YOUR BEST LIFE YET

Age Well
FITNESS

I0039940

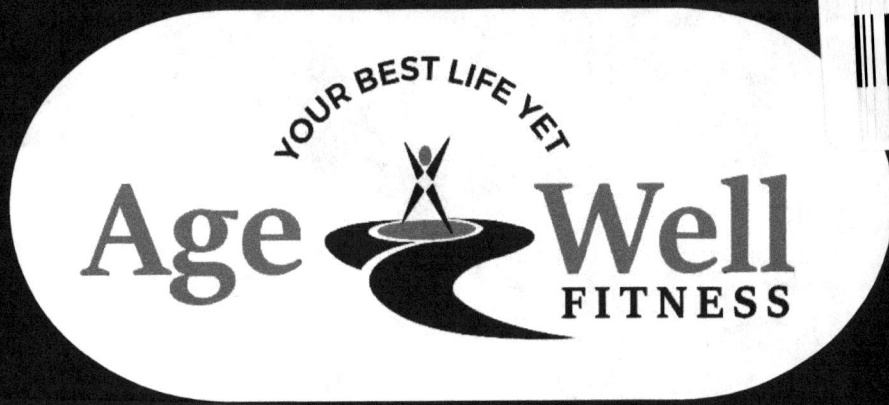

The Power of Small Steps
12 Monthly Challenges to Reset Your Health and Boost Your Well-Being

Use this workbook to explore wellness challenges and make sustainable wellness lifestyle changes, one month at a time. Whether you're just starting your wellness journey or looking for ways to stay consistent, this workbook will show you how focusing on one habit each month can lead to life-changing results. Let's commit to this together—one step, one day, and one challenge at a time.

By: Matthew "Max" Sturdivant a.k.a. Dr. Fitness | agewellfitness.org
Some images and content crafted with assistance from ChatGPT AI.

Table of Contents

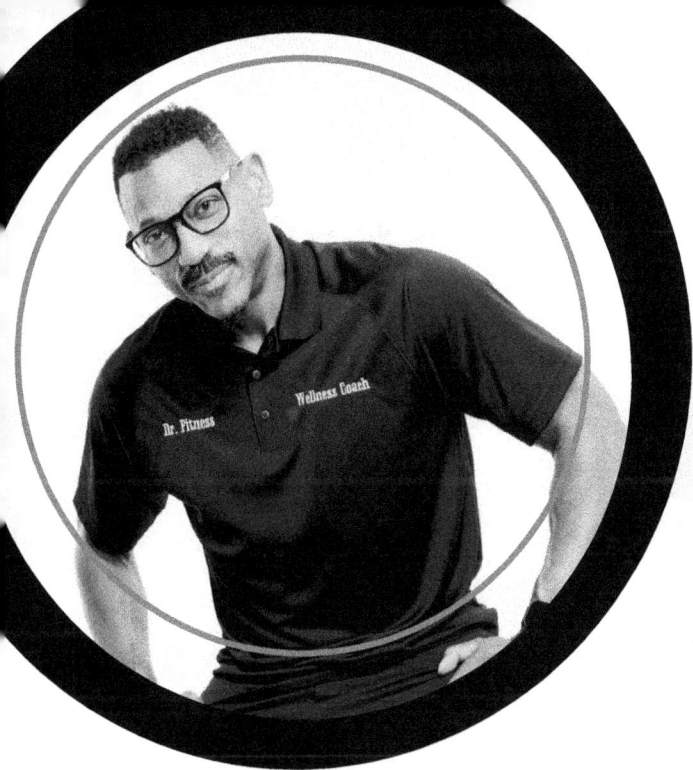

In today's fast-paced world, achieving and maintaining health often feels overwhelming. But what if the key to long-lasting well-being isn't a massive overhaul, but instead, small, intentional steps repeated daily? That's where my monthly health challenges come in. For many years, I've seen the power of these 30-day challenges transform lives—not by asking for perfection, but by encouraging progress. (The monthly challenges provide an opportunity to uncover unhealthy habits while sharing insights and strategies to modify daily habits that we are not aware are negatively impacting us).

While reading this book you will often notice I use the word WELLNESS. I believe it will be important to explore the definition of the word to better help you understand my choice of wellness over, let's say health or fitness.

Wellness typically includes several interconnected key items:

- **Physical:** Nourishing the body through exercise, nutrition, and proper sleep.
- **Mental/Intellectual:** Engaging in learning, problem-solving, and creativity.
- **Emotional:** Being aware of, accepting, and expressing feelings.
- **Spiritual:** Searching for meaning and higher purpose in life.
- **Social:** Connecting with others and engaging in meaningful community interactions.
- **Occupational:** Finding fulfillment and balance in work.
- **Financial:** Managing resources to live within one's means.
- **Environmental:** Fostering positive relationships between planetary health and human actions.

For the purposes of this book we will only focus on the first three of the 8 interconnected key items. I have noticed in my 30 year practice of supporting people on their wellness journey….if we properly focus on the first 3 we get amazing results and since the items are all so connected. We make significant progress on all 8 key points. For most of the clients and clinic patients I serve, accepting support with the first 3 are more socially accepted.

- Dr. Fitness (Max Sturdivant)

DISCLAIMER

This book is for informational and educational purposes only and is not intended to provide individualized medical advice, diagnosis, or treatment. The content within these pages is designed to support and encourage healthy habits but should not be considered a substitute for professional medical guidance.

Before beginning any new health or wellness program, including the challenges outlined in this book, consult with your physician or a qualified healthcare professional to determine what is appropriate for your individual needs. If you have any medical conditions, are pregnant, or are currently taking medications, seek professional guidance before making significant dietary or lifestyle changes.

If you experience any adverse effects or a medical emergency at any point during these challenges, discontinue immediately and seek medical attention. In case of an emergency, call your physician or dial 911.

By engaging in the activities and recommendations in this book, you acknowledge that you do so voluntarily and at your own discretion.

Building Healthy Habits, One Month at a Time

Health and wellness can often feel like an overwhelming mountain to climb. Between the busy pace of modern life and the constant bombardment of conflicting advice, it's easy to feel stuck or unsure of where to begin. But here's a secret: meaningful change doesn't require perfection or drastic measures. It starts with small, intentional steps—and the consistency to build those steps into habits over time.

That's the philosophy behind the 30-day health challenges in this book. Each month, we tackle a single health-focused habit. These challenges are designed to be approachable yet impactful, providing you with a focus for the month that creates lasting benefits for your mind, body, and spirit. The power of these challenges lies in their simplicity: you don't have to overhaul your life all at once. Instead, you're encouraged to dedicate 30 days to cultivating a specific habit, understanding its impact, and watching the ripple effect it has on your overall well-being.

Whether you're looking to improve your nutrition, strengthen your mental resilience, or break free from unhealthy patterns, this guide is here to support you. These challenges have been field-tested with real people—including my clients and myself—and they work. Along the way, you'll learn practical tips, encounter relatable stories, and gain insights that make even the toughest habits easier to master. And most importantly, you'll learn to trust the process and yourself.

You're not alone on this journey. Each challenge comes with encouragement, solutions to common obstacles, and ways to track your progress. By the end of this book, you'll have the tools and confidence to keep building healthy habits, no matter what life throws at you.

Let's get started—one month, one habit, and one step at a time.

How to Use This
Book

This book is designed to be your companion and guide as you embark on your journey to better health, one habit at a time. Each section focuses on a specific month and its corresponding challenge, providing everything you need to succeed. Here's how to get the most out of it:

1. **Start Anytime:** While the challenges are arranged month by month, you don't have to wait until January to begin. Choose the challenge that resonates most with you or aligns with your current goals and start from there.
2. **Set Clear Goals:** Before starting a challenge, take a few minutes to reflect on what you want to achieve. Whether it's losing weight, improving your mental health, or building a positive habit, having a clear goal will keep you focused.
3. **Engage Fully:** Each challenge comes with practical tips, action plans, and motivational stories. Commit to trying the suggestions and following through, even on tough days. Progress, not perfection, is the goal.
4. **Track Your Progress:** Use the included sample action plans, journal prompts, or a tracking app to monitor your journey. Noticing small wins along the way will keep you motivated.
5. **Adapt to Your Needs:** Life happens, and flexibility is key. If a certain aspect of a challenge doesn't fit your lifestyle, tweak it. The goal is to create a sustainable habit, not to feel restricted.
6. **Celebrate Your Successes:** At the end of each challenge, take a moment to reflect on your progress. Celebrate your wins, no matter how small, and use them as momentum for the next step in your journey.
7. **Build a Support System:** Invite friends, family, or coworkers to join you in the challenges. Sharing your journey with others can provide accountability, encouragement, and a sense of community.
8. **Revisit and Reinvent:** The challenges in this book can be repeated or customized as needed. Each time you revisit a challenge, you may discover new insights or opportunities for growth.

This book isn't just a guide; it's a toolkit for building a healthier, more intentional life. Use it as a resource to inspire positive change, and remember—every step forward is a step toward the best version of yourself.

Why 30-Day Challenges Work

30-day challenges are powerful because they focus on creating sustainable change without overwhelming you. They provide a structured, short-term commitment that makes trying something new feel achievable. Here's why they're so effective:

1. Focused Effort: Concentrating on one habit at a time allows you to give it your full attention. This focus increases the likelihood of success and prevents the burnout that often comes with tackling too much at once.
2. Achievable Timeline: A month-long timeframe is long enough to see tangible results but short enough to stay motivated. It feels manageable compared to indefinite commitments or large, abstract goals.
3. Habit Formation: Research shows it takes about 21 to 30 days to develop a new habit. These challenges guide you through that critical period, laying the foundation for long-term change.
4. Positive Momentum: Success in one challenge builds confidence and momentum for future changes. Completing a 30-day challenge proves to yourself that you can commit to and accomplish goals, inspiring continued growth.
5. Increased Awareness: By focusing on a single aspect of health each month, you become more mindful of your choices and how they affect your well-being. This awareness often spills over into other areas of your life.
6. Community and Accountability: Many challenges are more successful when done with others. Sharing progress, setbacks, and encouragement with a community or accountability partner can make the journey more enjoyable and rewarding.
7. Flexibility: Each challenge is adaptable to your starting point and lifestyle. You don't have to be perfect—the goal is progress, not perfection. Even small improvements can lead to meaningful results over time.

By breaking health and wellness into bite-sized, month-long challenges, you can create lasting change without feeling overwhelmed. These challenges serve as stepping stones to a healthier, happier you, proving that transformation is possible—one habit at a time.

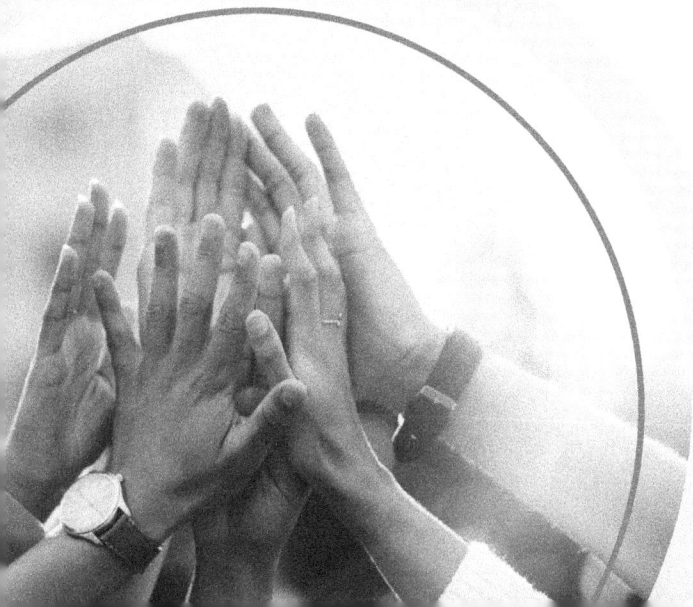

Themed Challenges
For Holistic Growth

Each monthly challenge in this book has been thoughtfully designed to address a specific aspect of health and wellness. Together, they form a holistic roadmap that nurtures your physical, mental, and emotional well-being. By focusing on one habit each month, you'll build a foundation of small, sustainable changes that add up to a healthier lifestyle.

Here's a closer look at the themes behind the challenges:

1. **Physical Health:** Challenges like "No Alcohol," "No Junk Food," and "Lose Belly Fat" prioritize detoxification, improved nutrition, and movement. These habits help strengthen your body, boost energy, and support overall vitality.
2. **Mindful Eating:** Themes such as "Eat Green" and "No Sugar" encourage you to rethink your relationship with food. These challenges teach balance, moderation, and the importance of nourishing your body with wholesome ingredients.
3. **Mental Clarity:** Challenges like "Mindful May" and "No Nicotine" emphasize mental resilience and focus. By letting go of distractions and harmful habits, you'll create space for mental clarity and peace.
4. **Hydration and Basics:** "Drink a Gallon of Water" highlights the foundational aspects of health that are often overlooked. Proper hydration impacts everything from digestion to energy levels, and this simple habit can work wonders.
5. **Behavioral Shifts:** Challenges such as "No Fast Food" and "No Soda or Juice" focus on breaking patterns that no longer serve you. By replacing these habits with healthier alternatives, you'll feel empowered to make better choices.
6. **Lifestyle Exploration:** The "No Meat April" challenge encourages curiosity and openness to trying new ways of eating. Even temporary shifts in diet can spark long-term discoveries about what works best for you.
7. **Body Awareness:** Themes like "Lose Belly Fat" combine nutrition, movement, and mindfulness to promote body awareness. By connecting with your physical self, you'll learn to appreciate and care for it in meaningful ways.

Consistency and Commitment: Every challenge underscores the importance of showing up for yourself. These 30-day commitments teach discipline and build confidence as you witness your ability to follow through on your goals.

Each month's challenge is more than just a task—it's an opportunity for growth and self-discovery. As you progress through the year, you'll notice the challenges working together to create a balanced and vibrant version of yourself. Whether you start at the beginning or jump in with the challenge that speaks to you most, you'll find that these monthly themes offer something for everyone.

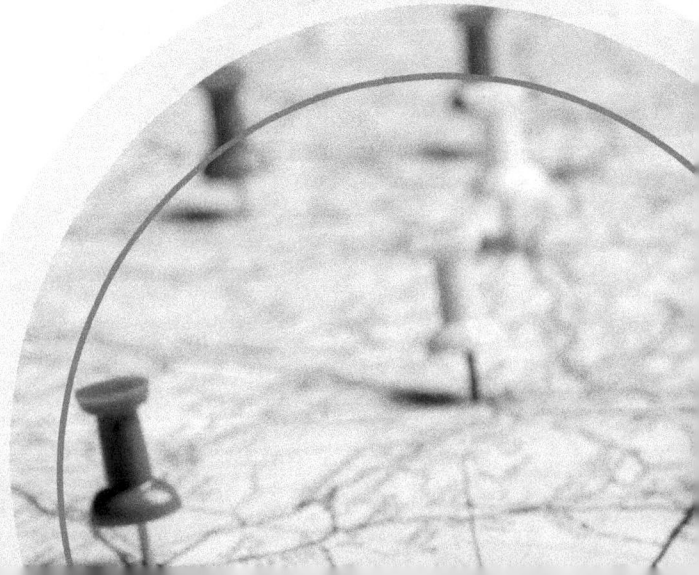

Turning Intentions Into
ACHIEVEMENTS

Setting clear, meaningful goals and tracking your progress are key to success in any challenge. These practices keep you focused, motivated, and accountable while providing a tangible way to measure your growth. Here's how to approach this process:

1 Set SMART Goals

A powerful goal is one that is Specific, Measurable, Achievable, Relevant, and Time-bound (SMART). Applying this framework ensures that your goals are clear and actionable. For example:

- Instead of saying, "I want to drink more water," set the goal: "I will drink 64 ounces of water daily during the Drink a Gallon of Water challenge."
- Instead of "I want to lose weight," set the goal: "I will lose 4 pounds by the end of the Lose Belly Fat challenge by eating balanced meals and exercising 3 times a week."

SMART goals help you stay on track and make it easier to celebrate your progress.

2 Break It Down

Large goals can feel overwhelming, so break them into smaller, manageable steps. For example:

- Weekly Milestones: "This week, I'll replace one soda per day with water."
- Daily Actions: "Today, I'll spend 10 minutes preparing a healthy lunch."

Small wins build momentum and give you confidence to tackle the next step.

3 Track Your Progress

Consistency is easier to maintain when you have a way to track your efforts. Use one or more of these methods:

1. **Journaling:** Reflect on your daily experiences. Write about your successes, challenges, and how you feel physically and mentally.
2. **Apps:** Download a habit-tracking app to log your progress. Many apps offer reminders, streaks, and graphs to keep you motivated.
3. **Visual Tools:** Use a wall calendar or habit tracker to mark each successful day. Seeing a visual record of your progress can be incredibly rewarding.

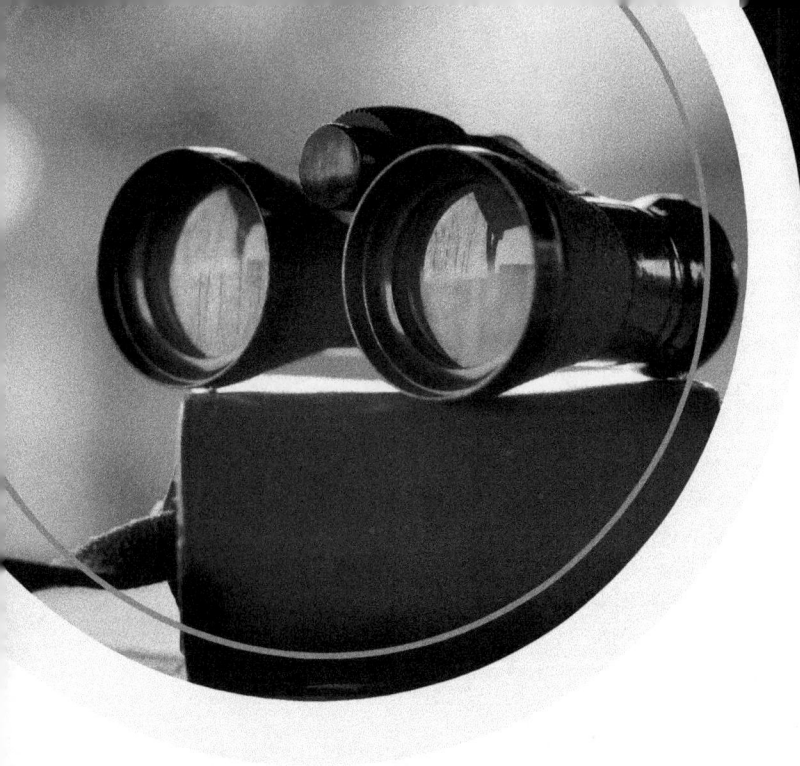

4 Celebrate Milestones

Acknowledging your progress keeps you motivated. Celebrate milestones such as completing a week without sugar or hitting a water-intake goal. Rewards don't have to be big—a relaxing evening, a small treat, or a heartfelt "I'm proud of you" can make a difference.

5 Reflect and Adjust

At the end of each challenge, take time to reflect on your experience:

- What worked well?
- What could you improve next time?
- How did this challenge impact your overall health and mindset?

Use these reflections to inform your goals for the next month. Remember, progress is not always linear, and adjustments are part of the journey.

By setting intentional goals and tracking your progress, you'll not only complete each challenge but also develop valuable skills that extend far beyond the pages of this book.

Why We Thrive
TOGETHER

Embarking on a journey to improve your health can sometimes feel isolating, but it doesn't have to be. The power of community support lies in its ability to provide encouragement, accountability, and shared experiences. When you connect with others who share similar goals, you create a network of motivation and resilience that makes achieving those goals easier and more rewarding.

Encouragement Through Connection

One of the greatest benefits of community is the encouragement it offers. Sharing your wins, challenges, and progress with others fosters a sense of camaraderie. Knowing that someone else understands your struggles can make even the toughest days feel manageable. A simple "You've got this!" from a friend or group member can be the boost you need to keep going.

Accountability for Success

When you commit to a challenge alongside others, you're more likely to follow through. Accountability can come from a workout buddy, an online group, or even a close friend who checks in regularly. This shared commitment creates a sense of responsibility, not just to yourself, but to the community. Knowing others are cheering you on keeps you focused and consistent.

Shared Experiences and Learning

Communities offer a wealth of shared knowledge. Members can exchange tips, recipes, and strategies that have worked for them, making it easier for you to navigate your own challenges. Whether it's discovering a new sugar-free dessert during the "No Sugar" challenge or learning stress-relief techniques during "Mindful May," these collective insights enrich your journey.

Celebrating Wins Together

Achievements feel even more significant when celebrated with others. Whether it's completing a week of healthy eating, running your first mile, or sticking to your hydration goals, sharing your victories inspires others and strengthens your own sense of accomplishment. Community members often become your biggest cheerleaders, creating a ripple effect of positivity.

How To Build Your
SUPPORT NETWORK

1. **Join a Group:** Look for local fitness classes, online forums, or social media groups dedicated to health and wellness challenges. These spaces are often filled with like-minded individuals eager to share their journeys.
2. **Invite Friends and Family:** Encourage your loved ones to join you in a challenge. Participating together creates a built-in support system and adds an element of fun.
3. **Use Technology:** Apps and social platforms can connect you with challenge groups and tracking tools. Many apps offer leaderboards, streak tracking, and messaging features to keep you engaged.
4. **Be a Supporter:** Offer encouragement to others in your network. Celebrating someone else's progress or helping them through a tough moment strengthens the bond and reinforces your own commitment.

The Ripple Effect

The support of a community doesn't just help you succeed—it creates a ripple effect. Your progress and positivity inspire those around you to take steps toward their own health goals. Together, you build a culture of wellness that extends far beyond individual achievements.

Community is a powerful force for change. By connecting with others, you'll find that every step forward becomes a little easier, every challenge a little less daunting, and every victory a shared celebration. Let's thrive together.

January

No Alcohol Challenge

Start the year with a clean slate by cutting out alcohol. Discover how abstaining from alcohol can boost your energy, improve sleep, and kickstart your fitness goals. Learn coping strategies for social events and create new habits that stick.

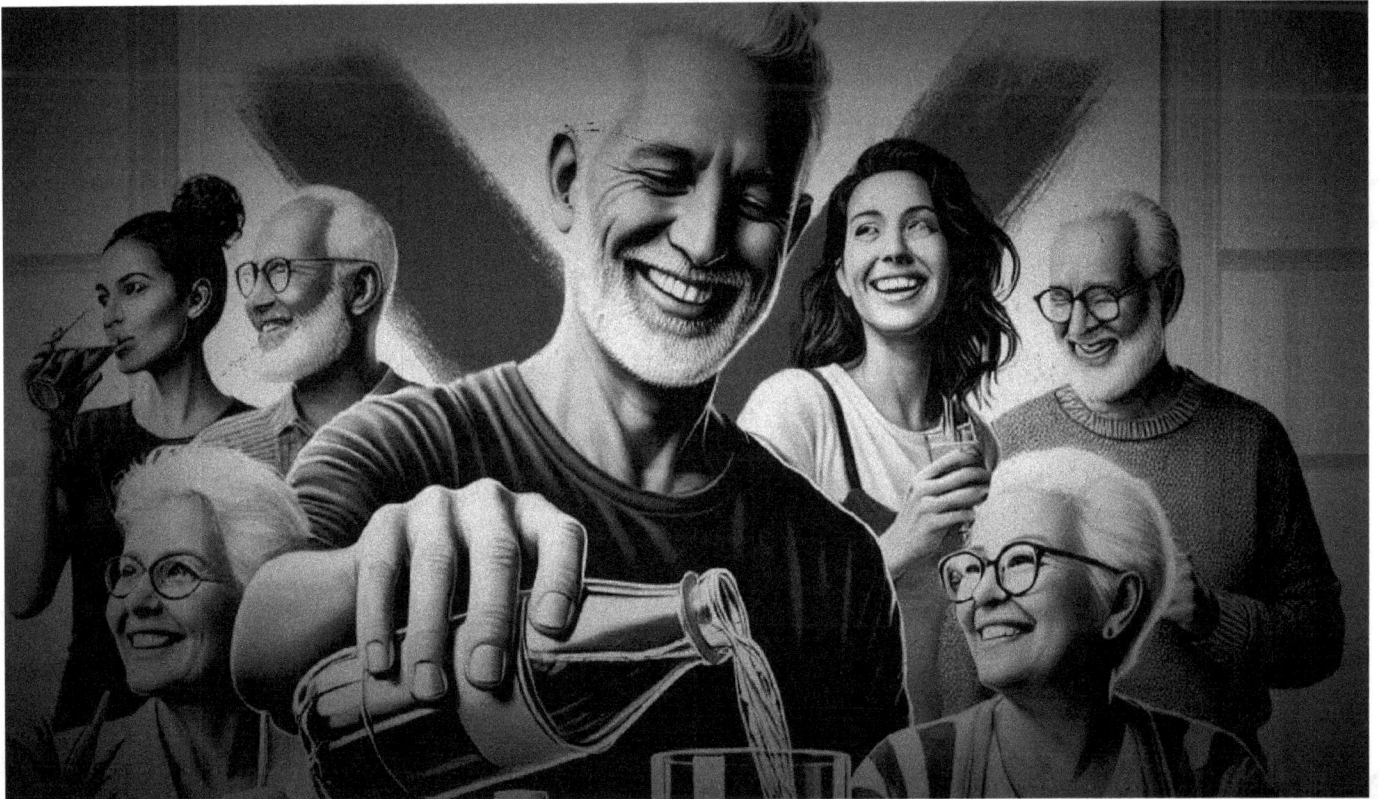

From Challenge to Change:
Real Participant Experiences

Real transformation happens when we take small, consistent steps toward better health. Each month, we challenge ourselves to build new habits, embrace positive changes, and support one another on this journey. But don't just take our word for it—hear from someone who has experienced the benefits firsthand. This testimonial highlights the real impact of this challenge and how it has helped others improve their well-being.

"My name is Carol, and I live in Orange Park, FL, with my daughter Susan. We're both educators, and like many families, we've faced challenges. I was deeply concerned about Susan's alcohol consumption, but I didn't know how to address it without starting a fight. Then I heard Dr. Fitness on the radio talking about the Dry January Challenge. His words stuck with me and my daughter—if alcohol isn't an issue, this challenge will be easy. But if it is, Dry January will highlight the problem and provide strategies or recommendations for professional care.

I decided to give it a try alongside my daughter, thanks to the encouragement and resources provided by Dr. Fitness. The workbook, along with the supportive structure of the challenge, made all the difference. Not only did Susan successfully complete the month, but she has now been sober for six months.

This experience has completely transformed our relationship—it's more positive, open, and supportive than it has been in years. I can't thank Dr. Fitness enough for the tools and guidance he provided through Dry January. It's no exaggeration to say it has changed our lives for the better."

— Carol, Concerned Mother & Educator, Orange Park, FL

The Hidden Benefits of an Alcohol-Free Month: What Science and Experience Reveal

January marks a fresh start—a time for setting intentions, reassessing habits, and prioritizing well-being. The No Alcohol Challenge isn't just about giving up alcohol for 30 days; it's about understanding what alcohol does to the body and mind while experiencing the powerful benefits of taking a break. Beyond the well-known effects like improved sleep and increased energy, here are deeper, science-backed benefits that may surprise you.

1. Your Gut Health Will Thank You
Alcohol disrupts the delicate balance of gut bacteria, often leading to inflammation, bloating, and poor digestion. Studies show that even moderate alcohol consumption can weaken the gut lining, contributing to issues like leaky gut syndrome and decreased nutrient absorption. Taking a break allows beneficial bacteria to flourish, improving digestion and overall gut health.

2. Mental Clarity and Emotional Resilience Increase
Most people expect to feel more energetic after quitting alcohol, but many don't realize how significantly it affects mental clarity. Alcohol slows cognitive function, disrupts neurotransmitters, and depletes essential vitamins like B1, which support memory and concentration. Even after just a week of sobriety, many report improved focus, reduced brain fog, and heightened problem-solving skills. Additionally, alcohol is a depressant, meaning abstaining can lead to improved mood stability and emotional resilience.

3. Your Immune System Strengthens
Alcohol weakens immune function, making the body more susceptible to colds, viruses, and infections. Studies suggest that after just three weeks without alcohol, immune cell production improves, strengthening your body's ability to fight illness. This means fewer sick days and more energy to tackle daily activities.

4. Blood Pressure and Heart Health Improve
Excessive alcohol consumption is directly linked to high blood pressure, irregular heart rhythms, and increased risk of cardiovascular disease. However, within just two weeks of abstaining, many people experience a noticeable drop in blood pressure, reduced inflammation, and improved circulation. Over time, this can lead to better overall heart health and reduced risk of stroke or heart attack.

5. Skin Rejuvenates and Hydration Levels Normalize
Alcohol is a diuretic, meaning it depletes the body's hydration levels, leading to dull skin, premature aging, and increased breakouts. Within 10 days of sobriety, skin hydration improves, elasticity returns, and a natural glow reemerges. Hydration also enhances nutrient delivery, making skin appear healthier and more vibrant.

6. Improved Metabolism and Weight Regulation
Alcohol is packed with empty calories and disrupts the body's ability to metabolize fat. When the liver is busy processing alcohol, it prioritizes this over burning stored fat, often leading to weight gain. Cutting alcohol for a month gives your metabolism a reset, allowing the body to focus on burning fat efficiently. Many people experience less bloating, better digestion, and even slight weight loss.

7. Social Awareness and New Coping Mechanisms
For many, alcohol is deeply ingrained in social settings and stress management. A 30-day break forces you to find new ways to unwind, such as meditation, journaling, or engaging in creative hobbies. It also brings awareness to how much social drinking influences habits, helping you make more conscious choices moving forward.

Final Thoughts: Beyond the 30 Days
Completing the No Alcohol Challenge isn't about eliminating alcohol forever—it's about discovering how you feel without it and reassessing its place in your life. Whether you decide to drink less, quit completely, or return with moderation, you'll walk away from this challenge with greater self-awareness, renewed energy, and a deeper understanding of how alcohol affects your health.

Are you ready to embrace the challenge and unlock these benefits for yourself? Your body and mind will thank you.

SMART *Goals*

Write your overall goal for this month's challenge.
- **S**pecific: What exactly will you do?
- **M**easurable: How will you track your progress?
- **A**chievable: How can you realistically achieve this goal?
- **R**elevant: Why does this goal matter to you?
- **T**ime-Bound: What is the timeframe?

_____

_____

_____

_____

_____

_____

_____

_____

_____

_____

_____

The beginning of a new year is the perfect time to reset, reflect, and prioritize your health. The 30-Day No Alcohol Challenge is designed to help you eliminate alcohol from your diet for one month, giving your body a break and allowing you to experience the benefits of sobriety firsthand.

Start the Year With a Clear
Mind and Body

Why Take the No Alcohol Challenge?

Alcohol is often seen as a harmless way to relax or celebrate, but its effects on the body and mind can be significant. Cutting out alcohol for 30 days can:

- Improve sleep quality, leaving you feeling more rested and energetic.
- Boost mental clarity and focus.
- Support weight loss by reducing empty calorie intake.
- Enhance liver function and detoxification.
- Increase overall energy and productivity.

Tips for Success
1. Set Your Intention: Write down your reasons for taking the challenge. Whether it's to improve your health, save money, or simply see how you feel without alcohol, having a clear intention will keep you motivated.
2. Plan for Social Situations: Let friends and family know about your challenge. Practice saying no politely and consider alternatives like sparkling water, mocktails, or herbal teas.
3. Track Your Progress: Use a journal or app to note how you're feeling each day. Documenting changes in your mood, energy, or sleep can help you stay on track.
4. Find a Buddy: Challenges are more fun with support. Invite a friend or join a group to share your journey.

Common Pitfalls and How to Overcome Them
- Cravings: Replace the ritual of drinking with a new habit, such as sipping tea or going for an evening walk.
- Social Pressure: Remember that your choice is about your health and well-being. A simple "No thanks, I'm trying something new" is often enough.
- Stress: Practice other stress-relief techniques like deep breathing, meditation, or exercise to handle tough moments.

Sample Daily Action Plan
- Morning: Reflect on your intention for the challenge.
- Afternoon: Drink plenty of water and enjoy a nutritious lunch.
- Evening: Replace alcohol with a healthy alternative and unwind with a calming activity, such as reading or yoga.

By the end of January, you'll likely notice a positive shift in your health and mindset. The best part? You might decide to continue this habit beyond the challenge—or use it as a springboard for other healthy changes in the months ahead.

January

- This is about clarity, not restriction. You're giving yourself the gift of better sleep, more energy, and mental sharpness.
- Your body starts healing right away. Even after just a week, your liver, brain, and immune system begin improving.
- Socializing without alcohol is freeing. You'll learn to enjoy moments without relying on a drink to relax.
- You're breaking the habit, not losing fun. True fun comes from experiences and connections—not alcohol.

Encouragement & Mindset Shift

Quitting alcohol for 30 days isn't just about what you're giving up—it's about what you're gaining. You're giving your body and mind a reset, allowing yourself to experience life without the haze of alcohol.

- Reframe the Challenge – Instead of thinking "I can't drink," try "I'm choosing to take care of my body and mind." This shift in thinking makes the challenge empowering rather than restrictive.
- Focus on How You Feel – You may notice better sleep, clearer skin, fewer cravings, improved mood, and higher energy levels. Keep track of these changes and remind yourself why you started.
- Cravings Are Temporary – When the urge to drink hits, pause for 10 minutes. Distract yourself with an activity, drink water, or remind yourself of your progress. Most cravings will fade quickly.
- Find a New Ritual – Many people associate alcohol with unwinding after a long day. Replace that habit with a new relaxing activity, such as sipping herbal tea, journaling, or taking a warm bath.
- Socializing Without Alcohol – If you're worried about social situations, plan ahead! Order a mocktail, bring a flavored seltzer, or tell friends you're on a personal challenge. You might be surprised at how supportive people are!

By the end of this challenge, you'll have a clearer mind, better health, and a sense of accomplishment. You might even decide that alcohol doesn't need to play such a big role in your life anymore.

Looking for Alcohol Alternatives?

Try These Instead!

Committing to 30 days without alcohol can bring powerful physical, mental, and emotional benefits. While changes may start subtly, over time, you'll notice improved energy, clearer thinking, and a stronger sense of well-being. Looking for a replacement? Here are some delicious alternatives to try.

If You Crave… Try This Instead!

Wine… Complex & Flavorful Alternatives
- Sparkling water with a splash of pomegranate or cranberry juice for tartness.
- Alcohol-free red or white wine for a similar taste without the effects.
- Hibiscus tea for a deep, slightly tannic flavor reminiscent of red wine.
- Grape juice mixed with soda water for a lighter, bubbly alternative.

Beer… Crisp & Refreshing Substitutes
- Alcohol-free beer for a familiar taste without the alcohol.
- Kombucha for a tangy, fermented kick.
- Sparkling water with lime for a refreshing, fizzy alternative.
- Ginger beer (non-alcoholic) for spice and depth without the alcohol.

Cocktails… Sophisticated Mocktails
- Club soda with fresh lime and mint for a simple, refreshing alternative.
- Fresh orange juice with soda water and a rosemary sprig for an aromatic drink.
- Cucumber and basil-infused water with a splash of lemon for a cooling effect.
- Cranberry juice, club soda, and a squeeze of lime for a tart, bubbly mix.

Whiskey or Dark Liquors… Bold & Warming Choices
- Black tea with a squeeze of lemon and honey for depth and warmth.
- Apple cider with cinnamon for a smooth, spiced alternative.
- Alcohol-free whiskey alternatives for a similar smoky, oaky experience.
- Warm vanilla almond milk with nutmeg for a creamy, cozy drink.

Margaritas or Tequila-Based Drinks… Tart & Citrus Alternatives
- Fresh lime juice with sparkling water and a pinch of sea salt for a refreshing, margarita-like experience.
- Alcohol-free tequila alternatives mixed with fresh citrus and soda water.
- Pineapple, lime, and coconut water for a tropical-inspired alternative.
- Iced herbal tea with lime and a splash of orange juice for a tart, fruity drink.

Nightcaps… Relaxing & Comforting Drinks
- Golden milk (turmeric, cinnamon, and warm milk) for a calming, sleep-friendly option.
- Chamomile or peppermint tea for a soothing end-of-day ritual.
- Tart cherry juice, which naturally promotes sleep.
- Warm honey-lemon water to wind down without the buzz.

Journaling Prompts
JANUARY

1 Reflect on your relationship with alcohol. What role does it currently play in your life, and how would you like to see that change?

_____

_____

_____

_____

_____

2 How do you feel mentally, emotionally, and physically after completing your first alcohol-free week? What differences have you noticed?

_____

_____

_____

_____

3 What new habits or rituals can you create to replace drinking? How can these habits better serve your overall health and well-being?

_____

_____

_____

_____

30 Days, 30 Wins: Your No Alcohol Challenge Calendar

Use the calendar below to mark off each alcohol-free day and see your progress build over the month. Each day, to jot down any physical or emotional changes you notice. Small shifts add up—by the end of the challenge, you'll have a clear picture of how going alcohol-free impacts your body and mind!

Sunday	Monday	Tuesday	Wednesday	Thursday	Friday	Saturday

February

No Soda or Juice Challenge

Reclaim your health by ditching sugary drinks. This chapter highlights the benefits of hydration, the hidden dangers of sugar, and how loving your body starts with mindful choices. Includes tips for making water exciting.

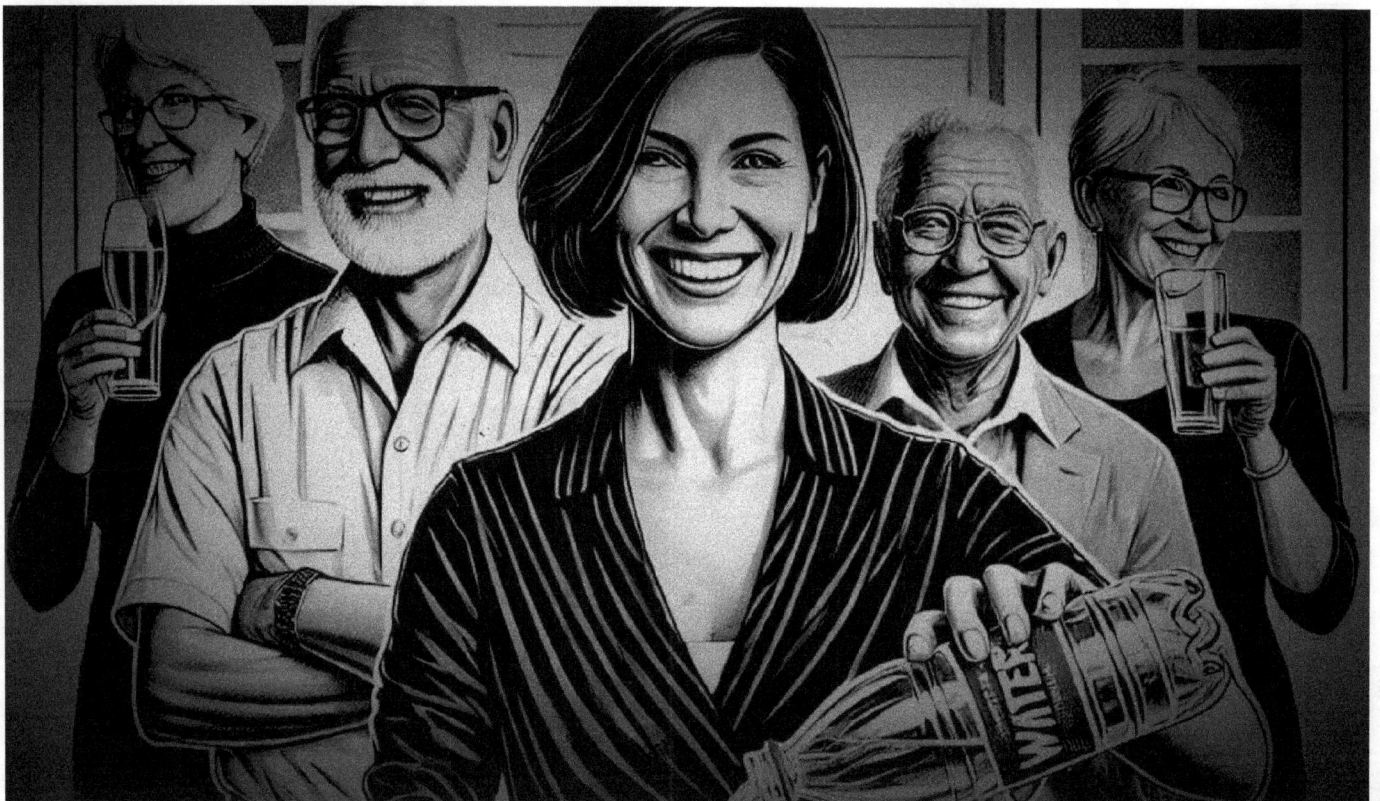

From Challenge to Change:
Real Participant Experiences

Real transformation happens when we take small, consistent steps toward better health. Each month, we challenge ourselves to build new habits, embrace positive changes, and support one another on this journey. But don't just take our word for it—hear from someone who has experienced the benefits firsthand. This testimonial highlights the real impact of this challenge and how it has helped others improve their well-being.

"As a lifelong soda lover, the February No Soda Challenge was a game-changer for me. Soda was tied to so many of my daily habits and childhood memories—it felt impossible to give it up. But when a friend encouraged me to join her and be her accountability partner, I decided to give it a try, and WOW, I had no idea how much I needed this challenge.

Dr. Fitness provided free resources that opened my eyes to the hidden dangers of drinking soda regularly, like how it contributes to tooth decay, bloating, and even disrupted gut health. This was a wake-up call. I realized I was addicted to soda, which explained why it was so hard to stop before.

The challenge taught me more than I expected. Not only did I quit soda for 28 days, but I also kept going and have now been soda-free for over a year! My teeth are healthier, my digestion has improved, and to my surprise, my waistline got smaller too.

This challenge changed my life, and I'm so glad I took the leap. If you're even thinking about cutting back on sugary drinks, I cannot recommend the February No Soda Challenge enough!"

— Jason S. - Soda Addict

Breaking Free from Sugary Drinks: The Science of Hydration and Health

Soda and sugary juices are more than just sweet treats—they're some of the biggest culprits behind energy crashes, metabolic disorders, and chronic inflammation. This month's No Soda or Juice Challenge isn't just about eliminating empty calories; it's about rewiring your body's relationship with hydration and experiencing how cutting sugar-laden drinks transforms your energy, metabolism, and overall health.

1. Blood Sugar Balance: A Key to Lasting Energy
Sodas and fruit juices contain high amounts of added sugars that spike blood sugar levels, leading to an inevitable crash. This rollercoaster of energy leaves you feeling sluggish, irritable, and craving even more sugar. Without these constant spikes and drops, your body can maintain steady energy levels, reducing brain fog and afternoon fatigue.

2. Liver Health and Detoxification
Did you know that fructose, the sugar found in sodas and many fruit juices, is processed almost entirely in the liver? Excessive consumption can lead to fatty liver disease, insulin resistance, and metabolic dysfunction. By eliminating these sugary drinks, your liver can focus on its natural detoxification process, improving digestion and overall metabolic function.

3. Weight Management and Metabolism Boost
Studies show that sugary beverages contribute significantly to weight gain. Unlike whole foods that provide fiber and nutrients, liquid calories bypass the body's natural satiety signals, making it easy to consume excess calories without feeling full. Cutting soda and juice helps regulate appetite, leading to better portion control and fewer cravings for processed foods.

4. Gut Microbiome Reset
Artificial sweeteners and high-fructose corn syrup disrupt the gut microbiome, killing off beneficial bacteria while allowing harmful microbes to thrive. The result? Increased bloating, digestive discomfort, and even weakened immune function. A month without sugary drinks gives your gut a chance to rebalance, improving digestion and reducing inflammation.

5. Oral Health: A Hidden Perk of Cutting Sugar
Soft drinks are one of the leading causes of tooth decay, as sugar feeds harmful bacteria that erode enamel. Even seemingly "healthy" fruit juices contain high acidity levels that weaken teeth over time. By eliminating these beverages, your teeth and gums will begin to repair, leading to fewer cavities and improved oral hygiene.

6. Reducing Hidden Additives and Preservatives
Beyond sugar, many commercial sodas and juices contain artificial flavors, preservatives, and phosphoric acid, which can deplete calcium and weaken bones over time. Opting for water, herbal teas, and naturally flavored beverages removes these hidden toxins, supporting bone health and long-term wellness.

7. Unlocking the Power of True Hydration
One of the most unexpected benefits of quitting sugary drinks is experiencing how real hydration feels. Instead of masking dehydration with sweet flavors, your body will begin to crave pure water, leading to improved skin elasticity, better digestion, and enhanced cognitive function.

Final Thoughts: Transforming Your Beverage Habits for Life
This challenge isn't just about avoiding soda and juice for 30 days—it's about redefining how you hydrate your body. By the end of the month, you'll likely notice improved energy, better digestion, and fewer sugar cravings. Whether you continue with water, herbal teas, or infused drinks, you'll have laid the foundation for a lifetime of smarter, healthier beverage choices.

Ready to take control of your hydration? Your body will thank you every sip of the way.

SMART *Goals*

Write your overall goal for this month's challenge.
- **S**pecific: What exactly will you do?
- **M**easurable: How will you track your progress?
- **A**chievable: How can you realistically achieve this goal?
- **R**elevant: Why does this goal matter to you?
- **T**ime-Bound: What is the timeframe?

_____

_____

_____

_____

_____

_____

_____

_____

_____

_____

_____

_____

_____

February is the month of love, making it the perfect time to focus on loving yourself by eliminating sugary beverages. The 30-Day No Soda or Juice Challenge encourages you to cut out these drinks for one month and experience how replacing them with healthier alternatives can positively impact your overall well-being.

Sweetened Beverages Out, Self-Love In

Why Take the No Soda or Juice Challenge?

Sugary drinks may be tasty, but their effects on your body and energy levels can be harmful. Giving them up for 30 days can:

- Stabilize blood sugar levels, reducing energy crashes.
- Support weight loss by cutting out empty calories.
- Improve dental health by lowering sugar exposure.
- Encourage healthier hydration habits.
- Reduce inflammation and its associated health risks.

Tips for Success
1. Find Alternatives You Love: Replace soda and juice with unsweetened teas, sparkling water, or infused water for variety.
2. Plan Ahead: Bring your favorite sugar-free beverages to work or social events to avoid temptation.
3. Set Mini Goals: Commit to drinking at least half your body weight in ounces of water daily.
4. Celebrate Non-Food Wins: Reward yourself with a non-food treat, like a relaxing bath or a new book, when you hit milestones.

Common Pitfalls and How to Overcome Them
- Cravings for Sweet Drinks: Gradually reduce sweetness by diluting juice with water before fully cutting it out. For soda, try sugar-free versions briefly before transitioning to healthier options.
- Social Pressure: Bring your own drink or confidently request water or unsweetened tea at gatherings.
- Boredom with Water: Experiment with flavors by adding fresh fruits, cucumber slices, or herbs like mint to your water.

Sample Daily Action Plan
- Morning: Start your day with a glass of lemon-infused water to boost hydration and digestion.
- Afternoon: Pack a reusable water bottle with fruit-infused water to sip throughout the day.
- Evening: Enjoy a calming herbal tea as a replacement for soda or juice.

By the end of February, you'll not only feel healthier but also more in control of your hydration habits. You may find that you enjoy the taste of water and other unsweetened beverages more than you expected. This challenge is a step toward a lifetime of self-love and healthier choices.

February

- Your body craves hydration, not sugar. After a few days, water will start tasting better, and your cravings will fade.
- Every soda-free day is a win. Skipping even one sugary drink prevents blood sugar spikes, crashes, and extra calories.
- You're retraining your taste buds. Once you cut out added sugars, naturally sweet foods will taste more satisfying.
- Replacing soda isn't deprivation—it's an upgrade. Your body will thank you with better digestion, energy, and hydration.

Encouragement & Mindset Shift

Cutting out sugary drinks is one of the fastest ways to improve your energy, balance your blood sugar, and reduce cravings. While the first few days might be tough, your taste buds and body will adjust.

- Your Taste Buds Will Change – The longer you avoid sugar-laden drinks, the more you'll enjoy natural flavors. After a few weeks, fruit and herbal teas will taste sweeter than ever.
- Cravings Mean You're Rewiring Your Habits – If you feel a strong craving for soda or juice, acknowledge it instead of fighting it. This is your body adjusting! Try sipping infused water, herbal tea, or sparkling water instead.
- Track the Benefits – Notice how you feel without sugary drinks. Is your energy more stable? Are you sleeping better? Do you feel less bloated? These small wins will motivate you to keep going.
- Stay Hydrated – Sometimes cravings for sweet drinks stem from dehydration. Keep a water bottle with you at all times and drink before you feel thirsty.
- Save Money & Your Health – Sugary drinks don't just affect your body—they also impact your wallet! Think of all the money you'll save by choosing water over expensive sodas and juices.

By the end of this challenge, you'll feel more refreshed, experience fewer cravings, and naturally gravitate toward healthier beverage choices.

Looking for Soda or Juice Alternatives?

Try These Instead!

Cutting out sugary and artificially sweetened drinks is one of the simplest yet most impactful ways to improve your health. Over the next 30 days, you'll focus on eliminating soda and juice while exploring natural, hydrating alternatives. Use this page to track your progress, discover new beverages, and reflect on how your body responds to this challenge.

Healthy & Refreshing Alternatives to Soda & Juice
One of the biggest obstacles in quitting soda or juice is finding satisfying replacements for the flavor, fizz, or sweetness you're used to. Try these alternatives to make the transition easier!

If You Crave… Try This Instead!
Soda… Sparkling Water & Natural Flavor Boosts
- *Sparkling water with fresh lemon, lime, or berries for natural flavor.*
- *Naturally flavored unsweetened seltzers for fizz without sugar.*
- *Club soda with mint and cucumber for a refreshing twist.*
- *Sparkling water with a splash of apple cider vinegar for a tart kick.*

Fruit Juice… Infused Water & Herbal Tea
- *Water infused with fresh fruit like strawberries, oranges, or basil.*
- *Herbal teas such as hibiscus, cinnamon, or berry for natural sweetness.*
- *Coconut water with a squeeze of lime for a lightly sweet alternative.*
- *Blended fresh fruit with water and ice for a juice-like refreshment.*

Energy Drinks… Natural Caffeine Boosts & Hydration
- *Green tea or matcha for a steady energy lift without the sugar crash.*
- *Yerba mate for a smooth, natural source of caffeine.*
- *Iced black coffee with cinnamon for a simple, sugar-free option.*
- *Coconut water with a pinch of sea salt for electrolyte balance.*

Sweet Tea… Natural & Refreshing Alternatives
- *Homemade iced tea with fresh lemon for flavor without sugar.*
- *Chilled hibiscus or peppermint tea for a refreshing, caffeine-free option.*
- *Unsweetened almond or cashew milk with cinnamon for a creamy, mildly sweet drink.*
- *Sparkling water with fresh ginger and lemon for a tangy, refreshing substitute.*

Sports Drinks… Natural Electrolyte Replacements
- *Coconut water with lemon and a pinch of sea salt for hydration.*
- *Watermelon juice with a dash of sea salt for a natural electrolyte boost.*
- *Homemade electrolyte drink with lemon, honey, and salt in water.*
- *Chia seed water with lemon for sustained hydration and energy.*

Every soda-free day is a win! Keep going and celebrate your progress—your body will thank you!

Journaling Prompts
FEBRUARY

1 What are your triggers for reaching for sugary drinks, and how can you address them?

_____

_____

_____

_____

2 How does your energy and mood change after a day of replacing sugary drinks with water or herbal tea?

_____

_____

_____

_____

3 What is one new healthy beverage you've enjoyed during this challenge, and why?

_____

_____

_____

_____

Tune In & Take Control:
Your 30-Day Beverage Awareness Tracker

This challenge is about becoming aware of your beverage choices and making healthier swaps. Each day, track your cravings, identify triggers, and note how you responded. At the end of each week, reflect on patterns and progress. By the end of 30 days, you'll have greater control over your habits, improved energy, and a refreshed approach to hydration!

Feel free to copy this page to track additional weeks and continue your progress.

Date	Time of Craving	What Triggered It?	How Did I Respond?	How Did I Feel After?
2/1	3:00 p.m.	Boredom, habit	Drank herbal tea	Felt satisfied

March

No Bad Carb Challenge

Explore the difference between good and bad carbs while embracing smarter food choices. This chapter dives into how refined carbs impact your body and provides a game plan for making healthy swaps that fuel your day.

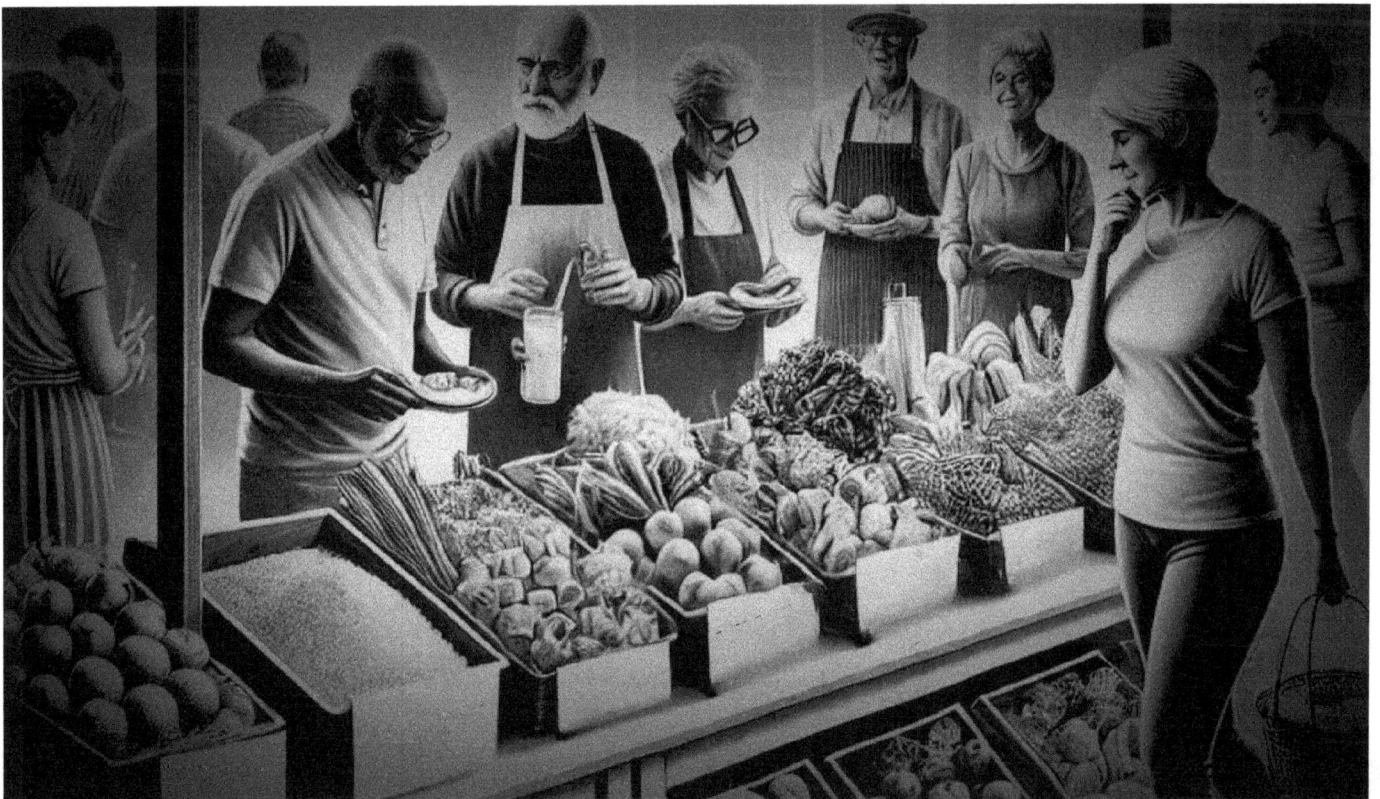

From Challenge to Change: Real Participant Experiences

Real transformation happens when we take small, consistent steps toward better health. Each month, we challenge ourselves to build new habits, embrace positive changes, and support one another on this journey. But don't just take our word for it—hear from someone who has experienced the benefits firsthand. This testimonial highlights the real impact of this challenge and how it has helped others improve their well-being.

"After spending 20 years in the Army, mandatory running took its toll on my knees and hips. When I retired, I was relieved to leave running behind, but over time, the hip and knee pain became unbearable. My doctor eventually referred me to Dr. Fitness, and I'm so glad they did.

Dr. Fitness introduced me to his March No Bad Carb Challenge, and it completely transformed my mindset about food. I always thought carbs were necessary with every meal, but through the challenge, I learned how to identify good carbs versus bad carbs and realized I had been sticking to bad ones for years. Dr. Fitness was compassionate yet firm—he had a way of pushing me toward change that always came from a place of genuine care.

The results were incredible! By cutting out bad carbs for just 30 days, I started reducing belly fat, inflammation and felt so much lighter overall, which significantly relieved the strain on my hips and knees. It's amazing how much of a difference diet can make. I couldn't be more thankful for Dr. Fitness and his guidance. His No Bad Carb Challenge didn't only help my body—it changed my lifestyle for good."

— Barb, 79, Retired Army Captain

The Truth About Carbs: Fueling Your Body the Right Way

Carbohydrates have long been misunderstood, with extreme diets either vilifying or glorifying them. But the truth lies in balance—not all carbs are bad. The No Bad Carb Challenge isn't about eliminating all carbohydrates; it's about breaking free from refined, processed carbs that cause energy crashes, weight gain, and long-term health risks. When you shift from quick-burning carbs to nutrient-dense alternatives, you unlock sustained energy, improved digestion, and enhanced brain function. Here's why this challenge is a game-changer for your health.

1. Stabilizing Blood Sugar: Ending the Energy Crash Cycle
Refined carbs—like white bread, pasta, and pastries—cause rapid spikes in blood sugar, leading to an inevitable crash. These fluctuations contribute to fatigue, mood swings, and increased cravings for more unhealthy foods. Replacing these with fiber-rich whole grains, vegetables, and legumes helps regulate blood sugar, providing steady energy throughout the day.

2. The Gut-Brain Connection: How Bad Carbs Impact Digestion
Your gut is home to trillions of bacteria that influence everything from digestion to mental health. Processed carbs, especially those high in sugar, feed harmful gut bacteria while starving the beneficial ones. This imbalance can cause bloating, inflammation, and even anxiety or depression. Choosing whole, complex carbs like quinoa, lentils, and sweet potatoes supports a thriving gut microbiome, improving digestion and overall well-being.

3. Reducing Inflammation and Chronic Disease Risk
Refined carbohydrates are linked to systemic inflammation, which plays a role in heart disease, diabetes, and autoimmune disorders. Eliminating processed grains and added sugars lowers inflammation markers in the body, reducing your risk of long-term health conditions and even improving joint pain.

4. Natural Appetite Control and Reduced Cravings
Ever notice how processed carbs leave you feeling hungrier, even after eating? That's because they lack fiber and essential nutrients, tricking your body into wanting more. Whole carbs digest slowly, keeping you full longer and reducing the likelihood of overeating. Foods like brown rice, beans, and fibrous vegetables provide steady nourishment and eliminate the need for constant snacking.

5. Boosting Brain Power with the Right Carbs
Your brain relies on glucose (from carbohydrates) for energy, but not all sources of glucose are created equal. Processed carbs deliver a short-lived surge, followed by mental fog and sluggishness. Whole-food carbs, like oats and berries, release glucose gradually, fueling focus and memory without the crash.

6. Fat Loss and Metabolic Efficiency
Refined carbs contribute to insulin resistance, making it harder for your body to burn fat efficiently. Cutting out bad carbs for a month allows your body to shift from storing fat to burning it for fuel. This challenge doesn't just promote weight loss—it improves metabolic health, making it easier to maintain a balanced weight long-term.

7. Unlocking the Power of Food as Medicine
When you swap out bad carbs for nutrient-dense alternatives, you're not just avoiding empty calories—you're nourishing your body with essential vitamins, minerals, and antioxidants. Instead of reaching for packaged snacks, this challenge encourages you to explore fresh, wholesome foods that work with your body instead of against it.

Final Thoughts: A New Relationship with Carbs
This challenge isn't about restriction—it's about empowerment. By eliminating bad carbs, you're giving your body a chance to reset, heal, and thrive. At the end of 30 days, you'll have a new appreciation for how whole foods fuel your energy, improve your digestion, and enhance your overall well-being.

Are you ready to break free from the cycle of processed carbs and embrace a healthier, more sustainable way of eating? Your body—and your future self—will thank you.

SMART *Goals*

Write your overall goal for this month's challenge.
- **S**pecific: What exactly will you do?
- **M**easurable: How will you track your progress?
- **A**chievable: How can you realistically achieve this goal?
- **R**elevant: Why does this goal matter to you?
- **T**ime-Bound: What is the timeframe?

_____

_____

_____

_____

_____

_____

_____

_____

_____

_____

March is a month of competition and excitement, making it the perfect time to channel that energy into tackling bad carbs. This 30-day challenge encourages you to eliminate refined and processed carbs while embracing whole, nutritious options. The result? Improved energy, better digestion, and fewer cravings for unhealthy foods.

Good vs. Bad Carbs:
Choosing Wisely

Why Take the No Bad Carb Challenge?

Not all carbs are created equal. While good carbs fuel your body and provide essential nutrients, bad carbs can lead to energy crashes, weight gain, and poor health. Removing processed carbs can:

- Stabilize blood sugar levels.
- Reduce unhealthy cravings.
- Promote steady energy throughout the day.
- Support weight management and gut health.
- Lower your risk of chronic diseases.

Tips for Success

1. Learn the Difference: Educate yourself on good vs. bad carbs. Whole grains, fruits, vegetables, and legumes are your friends; white bread, pastries, and sugary snacks are not.
2. Plan Your Meals: Prepare carb-friendly meals in advance to avoid the temptation of grabbing processed snacks.
3. Snack Smart: Keep healthy snacks like nuts, seeds, and fresh fruit on hand.
4. Hydrate: Drinking plenty of water can help manage cravings and improve digestion.
5. Incorporate Fiber: Foods high in fiber like lentils and broccoli will keep you fuller longer.

Common Pitfalls and How to Overcome Them

- Cravings for Processed Carbs: Gradually reduce bad carbs instead of quitting cold turkey. Replace them with whole grain or vegetable alternatives like quinoa or zucchini noodles.
- Social Settings: Plan ahead by eating a healthy snack before attending events where carb-heavy options may dominate.
- Feeling Deprived: Focus on the abundance of delicious whole foods you can enjoy instead of dwelling on restrictions.

Sample Daily Action Plan

- Morning: Start with a whole-grain oatmeal topped with fresh berries.
- Afternoon: Prepare a hearty salad with quinoa, vegetables, and a lean protein source.
- Evening: Opt for a stir-fry with brown rice and mixed veggies, seasoned with herbs and spices.
- Snack: Munch on a handful of nuts or fresh veggies with hummus.

By the end of March, you'll have a new appreciation for the power of good carbs and how they can fuel your body for success. Ready to bring your best game this month? Let's do this!

March

- This is about stability, not just weight loss. Less sugar and refined carbs mean fewer crashes, more energy, and balanced hormones.
- Whole foods keep you full longer. Instead of feeling deprived, you'll feel satisfied and fueled for longer periods.
- Cravings don't last forever. Within two weeks, your body will stop wanting refined carbs as much.
- You're not quitting carbs—you're upgrading them. Whole grains, fiber-rich veggies, and natural carbs give your body what it really needs.

Encouragement & Mindset Shift

Carbs are not the enemy—refined, processed carbs are. This challenge is about shifting from foods that cause energy crashes and cravings to whole, nourishing carbs that fuel your body.

- You're Not Cutting Carbs—You're Upgrading Them – Instead of white bread, pasta, and sugary snacks, you're filling your plate with fiber-rich grains, vegetables, and wholesome foods that keep you satisfied longer.
- Your Energy Will Stabilize – Refined carbs spike your blood sugar, leading to crashes and cravings. By swapping them for slow-digesting, whole foods, you'll experience consistent energy throughout the day.
- Cravings Mean Progress – If you're craving processed carbs, it's a sign your body is adjusting. Don't give in—reach for a healthy alternative like nuts, whole grains, or protein-rich foods. The cravings will lessen with time.
- Your Digestion Will Improve – Cutting processed carbs means less bloating and discomfort. Whole, fiber-rich foods help your gut function more efficiently.
- This Is About Long-Term Health – While weight loss may be a side effect, the real benefit is reducing your risk of diabetes, inflammation, and energy crashes.

By the end of this challenge, you'll have built a habit of choosing better carbs, feeling more satisfied after meals, and having steady energy all day.

Looking for Bad Carb Alternatives?

Try These Instead!

Carbohydrates are essential for energy, but not all carbs are created equal! Refined carbs and processed grains (like white bread, pastries, and sugary snacks) can cause blood sugar spikes, cravings, and energy crashes. This challenge focuses on eliminating bad carbs while embracing nutrient-rich whole foods that fuel your body for sustained energy and well-being.

Healthy & Satisfying Swaps for Bad Carbs
Cutting out bad carbs doesn't mean sacrificing flavor or satisfaction! Instead, try these nutrient-packed alternatives that keep you full, energized, and craving-free.

If You Crave… Try This Instead!
White Bread… Whole Grain, Sprouted, or Sourdough Bread
- Whole grain and sprouted breads contain fiber, vitamins, and minerals that refined white bread lacks.
- Sourdough is easier to digest and supports gut health due to its natural fermentation process.

White Rice… Quinoa, Brown Rice, or Cauliflower Rice
- Quinoa is packed with protein and fiber, making it a more balanced carb choice.
- Brown rice provides slow-releasing energy and keeps blood sugar steady.
- Cauliflower rice is a low-carb alternative for those looking to reduce overall carb intake.

French Fries… Baked Sweet Potatoes or Zucchini Fries
- Sweet potatoes are rich in fiber, vitamins A & C, and antioxidants.
- Baked or air-fried zucchini fries offer a crispy texture with fewer carbs and calories.

Chips… Roasted Chickpeas, Nuts, or Kale Chips
- Roasted chickpeas and nuts provide protein, fiber, and healthy fats, keeping cravings at bay.
- Kale chips are an easy, crunchy alternative full of vitamins and minerals.

Regular Pasta… Whole Wheat, Chickpea, or Zucchini Noodles
- Whole wheat pasta has more fiber and nutrients than traditional white pasta.
- Chickpea or lentil pasta boosts protein and keeps you fuller longer.
- Zucchini or spaghetti squash noodles offer a low-carb, veggie-packed alternative.

Sugary Pastries… Greek Yogurt with Nuts & Berries
- Greek yogurt provides protein and probiotics, while nuts and berries offer natural sweetness and crunch.
- Add cinnamon, cocoa powder, or a drizzle of honey for extra flavor without the sugar spike.

Sugary Drinks… Infused Water, Herbal Tea, or Sparkling Water
- Many sugary drinks contain hidden carbs and artificial ingredients.
- Instead, try fruit-infused water, caffeine-free herbal teas, or sparkling water for a refreshing swap.

Journaling Prompts
MARCH

1 How does eating whole, unprocessed carbs make you feel compared to refined ones?

_____

_____

_____

_____

_____

2 What challenges have you faced while eliminating bad carbs, and how have you overcome them?

_____

_____

_____

_____

_____

3 What are three new healthy carb options you can see yourself including in your regular diet?

_____

_____

_____

_____

Balanced Eating: Your 30-Day Smart Carb Journal

Use this log to track your meals, identify whether you're fueling your body with good carbs, and reflect on how satisfied you feel after eating. Each day, document your meals and snacks, note if they included whole, nutrient-dense carbs or processed, refined ones, and rate your satisfaction on a scale from 1 to 5. By the end of the challenge, you'll have a clear picture of how different foods impact your energy, cravings, and overall well-being!

Feel free to copy this page to track additional days and continue your progress.

Date	Meal/ Snack	Good Carbs? (Y or N)	Bad Carbs? (Y or N)	Satisfaction (1-5)	Notes (Cravings, Energy, Digestion)
3/1	Breakfast: Oatmeal	Y	N	5	Felt full until lunch - no cravings

5 - Very Satisfied   4 - Satisfied   3 - Neutral   2 - Slightly Unsatisfied   1 - Not Satisfied at All

April

No Meat Challenge

Discover the benefits of plant-based eating, even for just 30 days. Learn how to get enough protein, create balanced meals, and introduce variety to your diet while feeling energized and reducing inflammation.

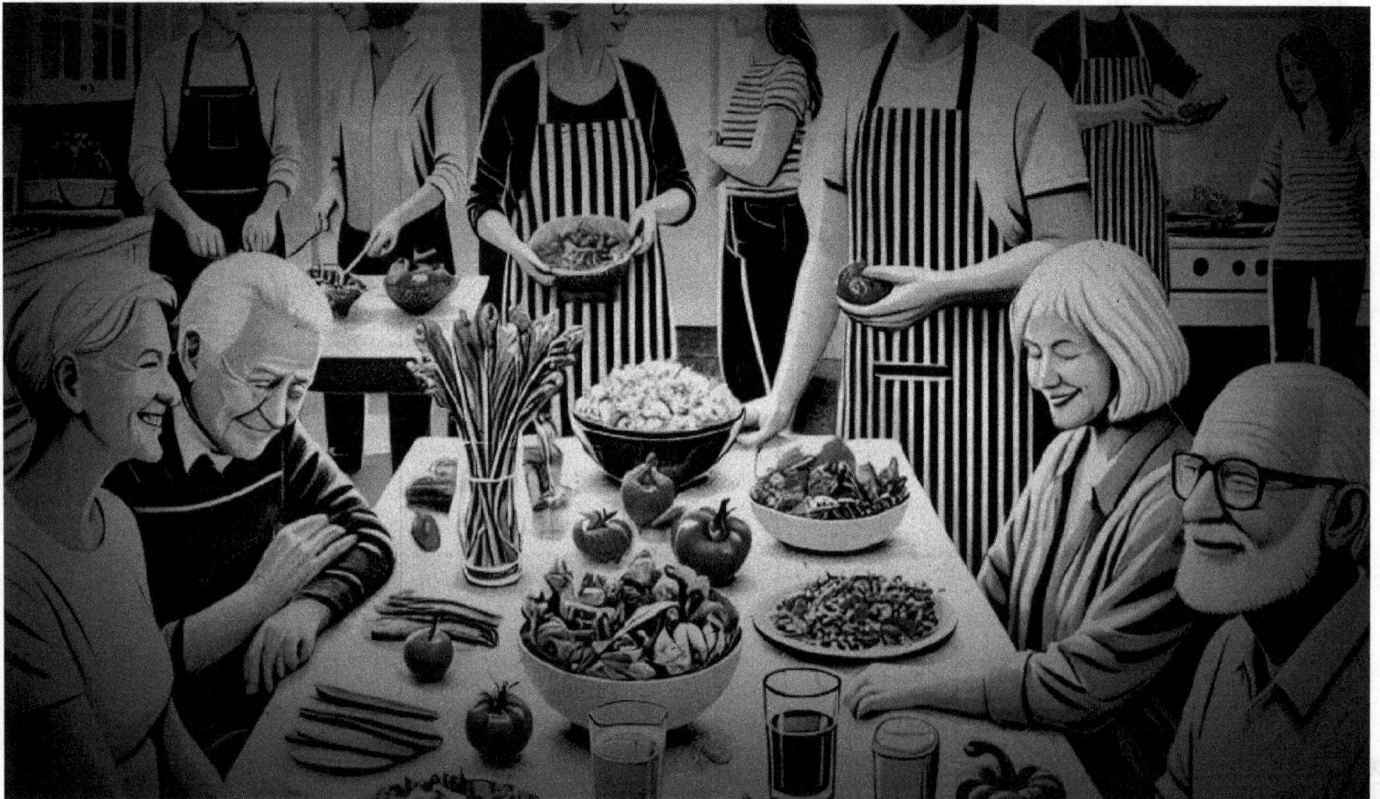

From Challenge to Change:
Real Participant Experiences

Real transformation happens when we take small, consistent steps toward better health. Each month, we challenge ourselves to build new habits, embrace positive changes, and support one another on this journey. But don't just take our word for it—hear from someone who has experienced the benefits firsthand. This testimonial highlights the real impact of this challenge and how it has helped others improve their well-being.

"Three years ago, I would have laughed if someone told me I'd thrive without meat in my diet. But then I was diagnosed with breast cancer and faced persistent issues like IBS, bloating, and digestion challenges. My oncologist recommended I work with Dr. Fitness, and that's when everything changed.

Dr. Fitness took the time to really understand my challenges and put together a personalized nutrition and exercise plan. He suggested the April No Meat Challenge as a starting point, explaining how processed meats and heavy meat consumption could negatively impact digestion and inflammation levels. I was skeptical—I was a daily sandwich eater! But with his guidance, I gave it a shot.

To my surprise, going meat-free for a month helped me feel lighter, more energetic, and significantly eased my digestive issues. The added fiber from plant-based alternatives improved my gut health and left me feeling better than I had in years. Most importantly, my body began to feel stronger and healthier.

That one-month experiment completely transformed my lifestyle. Not only am I now three years meat-free, but I'm overjoyed to share that my cancer is in remission today. I can't thank Dr. Fitness enough for the wealth of knowledge, encouragement, and support he provided. I truly believe the No Meat Challenge played a big role in my healing!"

— Monica W.

Going Meat-Free: Unlocking the Power of Plant-Based Nutrition

April is a time of renewal, making it the perfect month to reset your diet with the No Meat Challenge. Whether you're exploring plant-based eating for health, ethical, or environmental reasons, eliminating meat for 30 days offers a powerful opportunity to discover nutrient-dense foods, improve digestion, and reduce inflammation. But the benefits go far beyond what's on your plate—going meat-free can enhance your energy, mental clarity, and even long-term wellness.

1. A Boost for Heart Health
Diets high in red and processed meats are linked to an increased risk of heart disease, high cholesterol, and high blood pressure. Plant-based eating, on the other hand, naturally reduces saturated fats while increasing heart-healthy fiber. Swapping meat for legumes, whole grains, and leafy greens supports a strong cardiovascular system, helping regulate cholesterol and blood pressure levels.

2. Improved Digestion and Gut Health
Meat is harder to digest than plant-based foods, often leading to bloating and sluggish digestion. By cutting it out, you introduce more fiber-rich foods that support gut health, aid digestion, and keep bowel movements regular. A month without meat allows your gut microbiome to rebalance, improving nutrient absorption and reducing inflammation.

3. Lowering Inflammation and Disease Risk
While meat contains essential proteins, excessive consumption—especially of processed meats —can lead to chronic inflammation, increasing the risk of conditions like arthritis, diabetes, and autoimmune diseases. A plant-forward diet, rich in antioxidants and phytonutrients, fights inflammation and promotes healing from the inside out.

4. Sustainable Weight Management
Many meat products, especially processed varieties, are calorie-dense and high in unhealthy fats. Plant-based meals, on the other hand, are naturally lower in calories while being more filling due to their fiber content. This makes it easier to maintain a healthy weight without feeling deprived.

5. Unlocking Plant-Based Protein Power
One of the biggest concerns about eliminating meat is getting enough protein—but the truth is, plants are packed with it! Lentils, chickpeas, quinoa, tofu, and nuts provide all the essential amino acids your body needs, supporting muscle maintenance, metabolism, and overall strength.

6. Increased Energy and Mental Clarity
Heavy meat-based meals require more digestive energy, often leading to sluggishness after eating. In contrast, plant-based meals provide sustained energy and mental sharpness, helping you feel lighter, more alert, and more productive throughout the day.

7. A More Sustainable Future
Reducing meat consumption isn't just beneficial for your body—it's also a step toward a healthier planet. Meat production contributes significantly to greenhouse gas emissions, deforestation, and water depletion. Choosing plant-based meals, even temporarily, helps lower your carbon footprint and supports a more sustainable food system.

Final Thoughts: More Than Just a Diet Change
Eliminating meat for a month is about discovery—exploring new flavors, trying creative plant-based recipes, and understanding how your body feels when fueled by whole, plant-based foods. Whether you continue a meat-free lifestyle or simply reduce your intake in the future, this challenge equips you with the knowledge and experience to make informed dietary choices.

Are you ready to experience the benefits of plant-based living? Your body, mind, and the planet will thank you!

SMART *Goals*

Write your overall goal for this month's challenge.
- **S**pecific: What exactly will you do?
- **M**easurable: How will you track your progress?
- **A**chievable: How can you realistically achieve this goal?
- **R**elevant: Why does this goal matter to you?
- **T**ime-Bound: What is the timeframe?

_____

_____

_____

_____

_____

_____

_____

_____

_____

_____

_____

_____

April invites us to embrace renewal and growth, making it the perfect month to explore the world of plant-based eating. The 30-Day No Meat Challenge encourages you to eliminate meat from your diet and discover the variety, flavor, and health benefits that plant-based foods have to offer.

Explore the Benefits of a Plant-Based Lifestyle

Why Take the No Meat Challenge?

Going meat-free for 30 days can have significant health and environmental benefits, including:

- Lowering cholesterol and improving heart health.
- Reducing inflammation in the body.
- Supporting weight management by focusing on nutrient-dense, low-calorie foods.
- Enhancing digestion with fiber-rich meals.
- Contributing to a more sustainable planet by reducing your carbon footprint.

Tips for Success

1. Plan Your Meals: Look up plant-based recipes and prepare your meals in advance to avoid reaching for less healthy options.
2. Try Meat Alternatives: Experiment with tofu, tempeh, lentils, and beans to replace meat in your favorite dishes.
3. Focus on Whole Foods: Prioritize vegetables, fruits, whole grains, and legumes to maximize nutrition.
4. Explore Global Cuisines: Many cultures have delicious vegetarian dishes—try Indian dal, Middle Eastern falafel, or Mediterranean pasta with roasted veggies.

Common Pitfalls and How to Overcome Them

- Missing Meat: Satisfy cravings by incorporating umami-rich foods like mushrooms, soy sauce, and nutritional yeast.
- Lack of Protein: Ensure your meals are balanced by including protein-rich options like quinoa, chickpeas, and nuts.
- Social Situations: Bring a vegetarian dish to share or check menus for plant-based options when dining out.

Sample Daily Action Plan

- Morning: Enjoy a smoothie bowl topped with granola and fresh fruit.
- Afternoon: Savor a hearty grain bowl with quinoa, roasted vegetables, and a tahini dressing.
- Evening: Try a comforting lentil soup paired with whole-grain bread.
- Snack: Snack on hummus with carrot and cucumber sticks.

By the end of April, you'll have expanded your palate and gained a greater appreciation for plant-based eating. Whether you choose to stay vegetarian or reintroduce meat in moderation, you'll be equipped with the tools to make mindful dietary choices.

April

- This is an exploration, not a restriction. You're discovering new flavors, ingredients, and plant-based meals.
- Plants provide powerful nutrition. You're giving your digestion a break while still getting protein and essential nutrients.
- Protein comes from more than just meat. Beans, tofu, lentils, and nuts will keep you strong and satisfied.
- Every meal is an opportunity. You don't have to be perfect—just keep making progress.

Encouragement & Mindset Shift

Going meat-free for 30 days isn't about deprivation—it's about exploring new foods, flavors, and plant-based sources of protein. You'll feel lighter, experience better digestion, and expand your meal options in ways you never imagined.

- You're Not Losing Protein—You're Finding New Sources – Beans, lentils, quinoa, nuts, and tofu all provide protein while delivering essential vitamins and minerals.
- Your Body Will Feel the Difference – Cutting back on meat can lead to less bloating, more energy, and improved digestion. Many people also notice clearer skin and better sleep.
- Mindset Shift: Think Addition, Not Restriction – Instead of focusing on what you can't eat, get excited about trying new plant-based meals, spices, and ingredients.
- You Can Still Get Full and Satisfied – Many plant-based foods are packed with fiber, which means you'll feel full longer.
- Every Meal Is a Learning Experience – This isn't just about 30 days—it's about finding plant-based meals you love that you can continue to enjoy after the challenge.

By the end of this challenge, you'll have a new appreciation for plant-based eating, better digestion, and a list of new favorite meals!

Looking for Meat-Free Alternatives?

Try These Instead!

Eliminating meat for 30 days doesn't mean sacrificing protein, flavor, or satisfaction. By choosing nutrient-dense, plant-based alternatives, you can still enjoy hearty, protein-packed meals while exploring new ingredients. Here are some delicious meat-free replacements to help you stay on track with the challenge.

If You Crave... Try This Instead!

Chicken... Protein-Rich & Versatile Substitutes
- Tofu (firm or extra firm) marinated and grilled for a similar texture.
- Tempeh for a hearty, nutty-flavored alternative with extra protein.
- Jackfruit (unripe) for a shredded, chicken-like consistency in tacos and sandwiches.
- Chickpeas in stir-fries, salads, or mashed for a creamy texture.

Beef... Hearty & Flavorful Replacements
- Lentils cooked with smoked paprika for a ground beef alternative in tacos or pasta.
- Mushrooms (portobello or cremini) for a rich, umami-packed meat replacement.
- Black beans or kidney beans for a filling, meaty texture in stews and chili.
- Walnut and mushroom mix for a plant-based ground "meat" substitute.

Pork... Savory, Smoky Options
- Seitan (wheat-based protein) for a chewy, meat-like texture in stir-fries.
- Smoked tofu or tempeh for bacon-like flavor in sandwiches and salads.
- Eggplant marinated and grilled for a smoky, tender alternative.
- Coconut bacon (thinly sliced coconut, baked with tamari and liquid smoke) for a crispy topping.

Fish & Seafood... Light Yet Satisfying Swaps
- Hearts of palm for a flaky, fish-like texture in ceviche or "crab" cakes.
- Nori seaweed and chickpeas blended for a plant-based tuna salad.
- Marinated tofu or tempeh with lemon and Old Bay seasoning for a seafood-inspired flavor.
- Mushrooms or artichokes as substitutes for scallops or calamari.

Meaty Burgers... Juicy & Filling Alternatives
- Black bean and quinoa patties for a high-protein, hearty burger.
- Beyond Meat or Impossible Burger for a plant-based burger that mimics beef.
- Portobello mushroom caps grilled and topped with seasonings for a juicy bite.
- Lentil and walnut patties for a rich, savory option.

Deli Meats... Sandwich-Friendly Swaps
- Hummus, avocado, or mashed chickpeas for creamy, protein-rich spreads.
- Smoked tempeh or tofu for sandwich layers with depth of flavor.
- Roasted red peppers and eggplant for a satisfying, savory bite.
- Vegan deli slices (store-bought) for a convenient grab-and-go alternative.

Meat-Based Broths... Flavorful Plant-Based Stocks
- Vegetable broth enhanced with miso paste for extra umami.
- Mushroom broth for a deep, rich flavor in soups and stews.
- Coconut milk with spices for a creamy, flavorful soup base.
- Roasted garlic and onion-infused broth for depth in sauces and gravies.

Journaling Prompts
APRIL

1 How does eating plant-based meals make you feel physically and emotionally?

_____

_____

_____

_____

2 What are the most creative or flavorful plant-based meals you've tried during this challenge?

_____

_____

_____

_____

3 How has this challenge changed your perspective on food and its impact on the environment?

_____

_____

_____

_____

Plant-Powered Tracker: 30 Days of Meat-Free Meals

Use this tracker to log your daily meat-free meals and explore new plant-based ingredients and recipes. Each day, check off your meals, take note of any new foods you tried, and reflect on how you feel—whether it's improved energy, better digestion, or new cravings. By the end of 30 days, you'll have a better understanding of plant-based eating and a list of delicious, meat-free meals to keep in your routine!

Feel free to copy this page to track additional weeks and continue your progress.

Date	B-fast	Lunch	Dinner	Snacks	New Ingredients or Recipes Tried	Notes (Energy, Digestion, Cravings)
4/1	✔	✔	✗	✔	Tofu Scramble	Craved meat at dinner, will adjust portion sizes

May

Mindful May Challenge

Shift your mindset with mindfulness. From mindful eating to stress management, this chapter encourages you to slow down, focus on the present, and build emotional resilience.

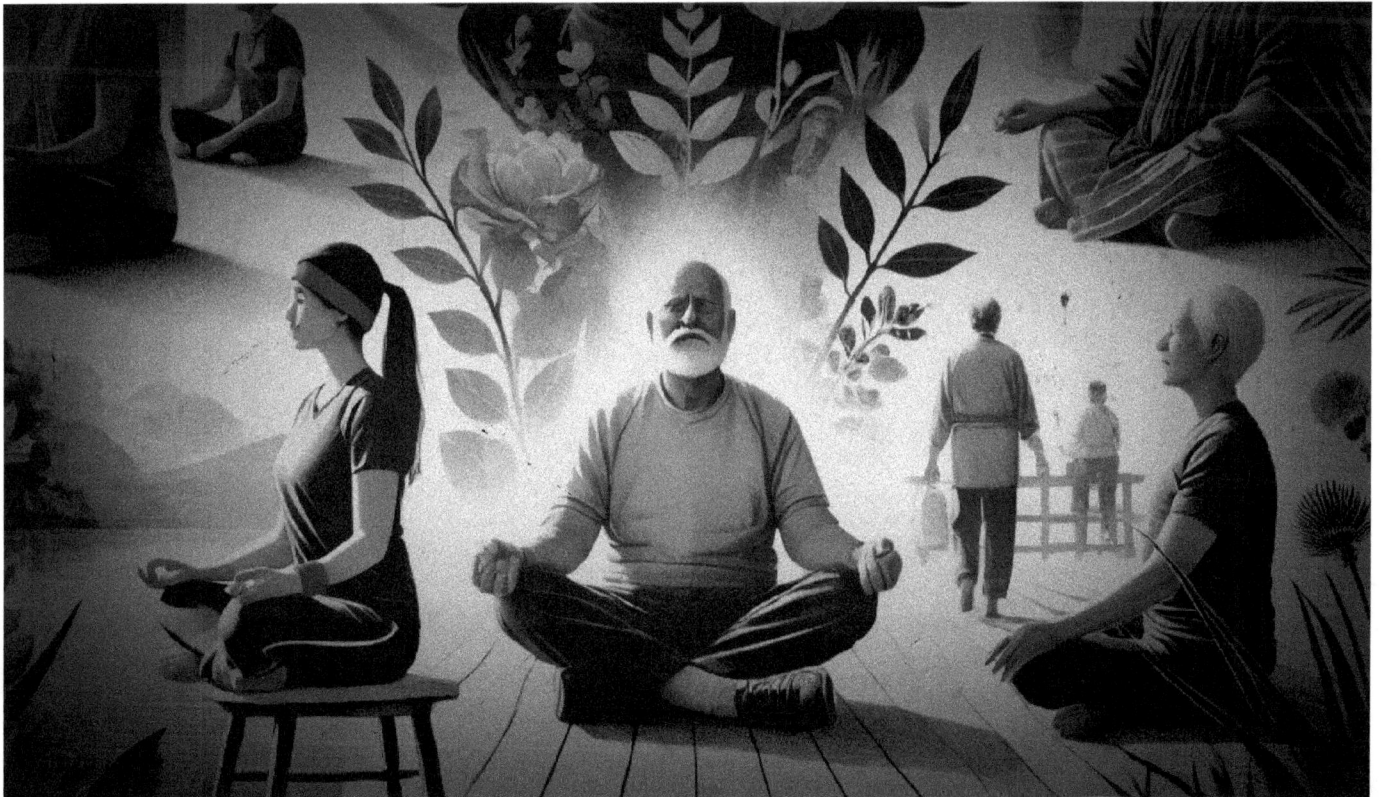

From Challenge to Change:
Real Participant Experiences

Real transformation happens when we take small, consistent steps toward better health. Each month, we challenge ourselves to build new habits, embrace positive changes, and support one another on this journey. But don't just take our word for it—hear from someone who has experienced the benefits firsthand. This testimonial highlights the real impact of this challenge and how it has helped others improve their well-being.

"I can't recommend the Mindful May Challenge enough! Before starting, I was dealing with poor sleep, elevated blood pressure, and overwhelming anxiety from work. Thanks to the incredible support from Dr. Fitness, the challenge was easy to follow and made such a difference in my life!

Not only did I sleep better, but my blood pressure also dropped, and my anxiety significantly decreased. The challenge introduced me to mindfulness practices that helped me regulate my response to stress, leaving me feeling more patient, emotionally balanced, and clear-headed.

If you're struggling with anxiety or difficulty sleeping, I strongly encourage you to try the Mindful May Challenge. It's been a game-changer for my well-being!"

— Jerrian

The Science of Mindfulness: How Awareness Transforms Health and Well-Being

In a world that constantly demands our attention, mindfulness offers a powerful antidote to stress, overwhelm, and disconnection. The Mindful May Challenge isn't just about meditation—it's about cultivating a deeper presence in daily life, training your mind to focus, and learning how to truly listen to your body. Practicing mindfulness for 30 days can significantly impact mental clarity, emotional balance, and even physical health in ways you might not expect.

1. The Mind-Body Connection: How Mindfulness Supports Physical Health
Mindfulness isn't just a mental exercise; it has profound physiological effects. Studies show that mindful practices can lower blood pressure, reduce chronic pain, and even boost immune function. When you slow down and bring awareness to your body, your nervous system shifts from a stressed state (fight-or-flight) to a relaxed state (rest-and-digest), allowing for healing and repair.

2. Stress Reduction and Emotional Resilience
One of the most well-documented benefits of mindfulness is its ability to lower cortisol, the stress hormone. Chronic stress is linked to inflammation, poor sleep, and weight gain, but mindfulness teaches you how to regulate your response to stress. With regular practice, you'll find yourself reacting to challenges with more patience, emotional balance, and clarity.

3. Improved Digestion Through Mindful Eating
How often do you eat while scrolling through your phone or watching TV? Mindless eating can lead to overeating, poor digestion, and reduced satisfaction with meals. Mindful eating encourages you to slow down, chew thoroughly, and truly taste your food, leading to better digestion, improved nutrient absorption, and a healthier relationship with food.

4. Boosting Focus and Cognitive Function
The ability to concentrate is a skill that can be strengthened, just like a muscle. Mindfulness trains the brain to stay present, improving attention span, memory, and decision-making. Even just 10 minutes of mindfulness practice a day can increase gray matter in the brain, enhancing cognitive function and mental sharpness.

5. Enhancing Sleep Quality
Mindfulness helps regulate the nervous system, making it easier to transition into deep, restorative sleep. If racing thoughts keep you up at night, practicing mindfulness can calm the mind and promote better sleep patterns. Techniques like body scans and breathwork are especially effective for improving sleep quality.

6. Strengthening Relationships Through Presence
Being truly present in conversations—without distractions—can deepen relationships and improve communication. Mindfulness encourages active listening, empathy, and non-reactivity, fostering stronger connections with loved ones, colleagues, and even strangers.

7. A Gateway to Greater Self-Awareness
Perhaps the most profound benefit of mindfulness is the ability to observe thoughts and emotions without being consumed by them. This awareness creates space for intentional choices rather than reactive behaviors, allowing you to align more closely with your values, goals, and authentic self.

Final Thoughts: A Lifelong Skill, Not Just a Challenge
Mindfulness isn't something to check off a to-do list—it's a way of approaching life with greater awareness, gratitude, and presence. As you move through the Mindful May Challenge, you'll begin to notice small but powerful shifts in how you experience the world. Whether it's feeling more peaceful, less reactive, or more attuned to your body's needs, mindfulness is a lifelong practice that brings lasting transformation.

Are you ready to quiet the noise, tune into yourself, and experience the power of mindfulness? Your body and mind will thank you.

SMART *Goals*

Write your overall goal for this month's challenge.
- **S**pecific: What exactly will you do?
- **M**easurable: How will you track your progress?
- **A**chievable: How can you realistically achieve this goal?
- **R**elevant: Why does this goal matter to you?
- **T**ime-Bound: What is the timeframe?

_____

_____

_____

_____

_____

_____

_____

_____

_____

_____

_____

_____

May is a time to pause and reconnect with your inner self. The 30-Day Mindful May Challenge focuses on practicing mindfulness to reduce stress, enhance mental clarity, and foster a deeper sense of calm and gratitude. By dedicating just a few moments each day to being fully present, you'll discover the profound benefits mindfulness can bring to your life.

Embrace the Present, Reduce Stress,
And Find Inner Peace

Why Take the Mindful May Challenge?

Mindfulness is a powerful tool for improving overall well-being. Committing to this challenge can:

- Reduce stress and anxiety by anchoring you in the present moment.
- Improve focus and productivity through greater mental clarity.
- Foster emotional regulation and resilience.
- Enhance relationships by promoting active listening and empathy.
- Cultivate gratitude and joy in everyday life.

Tips for Success
1. Start Small: Begin with just 5 minutes of mindfulness practice per day and gradually increase as you feel comfortable.
2. Create a Dedicated Space: Set up a quiet, clutter-free area in your home for mindfulness activities like meditation or journaling.
3. Incorporate It Into Your Day: Practice mindfulness during routine activities, such as eating, walking, or brushing your teeth.
4. Use Guided Resources: Apps, podcasts, or YouTube videos can provide helpful guided meditations to support your journey.

Common Pitfalls and How to Overcome Them
- Difficulty Staying Focused: Acknowledge when your mind wanders and gently bring your attention back to the present moment.
- Skipping Days: Set reminders or schedule your mindfulness practice at the same time each day to build consistency.
- Impatience: Remember that mindfulness is a practice. The benefits will become more noticeable over time with consistent effort.

Sample Daily Action Plan
- Morning: Start your day with a 5-minute meditation or deep-breathing exercise.
- Afternoon: Take a mindful walk, focusing on the sights, sounds, and sensations around you.
- Evening: Reflect on three things you're grateful for and journal your thoughts before bed.

By the end of May, you'll have cultivated a habit of mindfulness that supports your mental and emotional well-being. You'll find yourself approaching life's challenges with greater ease and appreciation for the present moment.

May

- Every moment is an opportunity to be present. You don't need hours of meditation—just pause and breathe.
- Distraction is normal, but awareness brings power. The more you notice your mind wandering, the easier it becomes to refocus.
- You can't control everything, but you can control your response. Mindfulness helps you react with clarity instead of stress.
- Small daily shifts create lasting change. One mindful action a day leads to less anxiety, better focus, and more joy.

Encouragement & Mindset Shift

Life moves fast, and we often operate on autopilot. This challenge is about slowing down, paying attention, and learning to be present in your daily experiences.

- Mindfulness Isn't About Perfection – Your mind will wander, and that's okay. The key is to gently bring yourself back to the present.
- You'll Feel More in Control – Instead of reacting impulsively, mindfulness helps you pause, reflect, and respond with intention.
- Less Stress, More Joy – Mindfulness reduces anxiety and overthinking, helping you fully enjoy the moment. Small Shifts Make a Big Impact – You don't need to meditate for hours—just taking deep breaths, eating without distractions, or focusing on your surroundings can create change.
- Life Becomes More Meaningful – When you stop rushing and start noticing, you'll find beauty and gratitude in everyday moments.

By the end of this challenge, you'll feel more centered, present, and in control of your emotions and actions.

Looking for Presence-Boosting Alternatives?
Try These Instead!

Breaking free from autopilot and distraction starts with small, intentional shifts. Instead of reacting out of habit, choose a mindful alternative that brings you back to the present. Try these simple swaps to cultivate awareness and presence in your daily life.

If You Crave… Try This Instead!
Distraction (Mindless Scrolling, TV Bingeing)… Intentional Connection
- Set a 5-minute timer before opening social media to check in with how you're feeling.
- Replace screen time with a mindful activity like journaling, coloring, or stretching.
- Call or text a friend instead of endlessly scrolling.
- Swap background noise for silence or nature sounds to increase awareness.

Autopilot Routines… Conscious Awareness
- Brush your teeth, shower, or do dishes with full attention, noticing each sensation.
- Take a different route on your walk or drive and observe new details.
- Pause before eating and take one deep breath to fully experience the flavors.
- Start a daily gratitude check-in—notice three things you're grateful for each morning.

Overthinking & Mental Clutter… Present Moment Awareness
- When your mind races, focus on your breath, counting each inhale and exhale.
- Label your thoughts: Is this a worry, a memory, or a future plan? Then gently return to now.
- Use grounding techniques like noticing five things you see, hear, and feel around you.
- Swap mental spirals for a mindful walk, paying attention to each step and breath.

Multitasking… Single-Task Focus
- Choose one task at a time and commit fully—whether it's eating, working, or talking to someone.
- Set a timer for deep focus, working undistracted for 20 minutes before taking a mindful break.
- Instead of checking emails while eating, savor your food without distractions.
- Replace rushing through tasks with intentional pauses between each activity.

Emotional Reactivity… Thoughtful Response
- Before reacting, pause and take three deep breaths. Notice how your body feels.
- When feeling overwhelmed, step outside or move your body to shift your state.
- If irritation arises, label the emotion rather than acting on it immediately.
- Swap judgment for curiosity—ask yourself, "What am I really feeling?"

Journaling Prompts
MAY

1 What is one moment today when you felt fully present and mindful? How did it feel?

_____

_____

_____

_____

_____

2 How does practicing mindfulness impact your stress levels or relationships?

_____

_____

_____

_____

_____

3 What are three simple ways you can incorporate mindfulness into your daily routine?

_____

_____

_____

_____

Your Mindfulness Tracker:
Cultivating Awareness Daily

This challenge is all about bringing more awareness and presence into your daily life. Each day, use this journal to record how you practiced mindfulness—whether through meditation, mindful eating, a nature walk, or simply taking a few deep breaths. Then, reflect on how present you felt on a scale from 1 to 5 and jot down any insights. By the end of the month, you'll have a clearer understanding of what mindfulness techniques work best for you and how they impact your well-being!

Feel free to copy this page to track additional weeks and continue your progress.

Date	Mindfulness Practice (Meditation, Walk, Etc.)	How Present Did I Feel (1 to 5)?	Reflections, Thoughts, Feelings, Insights
5/1	5-minute breathing meditation	4 - felt calm but distracted	Struggled at first but felt more relaxed by the end

5 - Fully Present **4** - Mostly Present **3** - Somewhat Present **2** - Barely Present **1** - Not Present at All

June

No Junk Food Challenge

Unpack the hidden ingredients in processed foods and learn how to replace them with nutritious alternatives. This chapter includes snack ideas, meal prep tips, and guidance on breaking the junk food cycle.

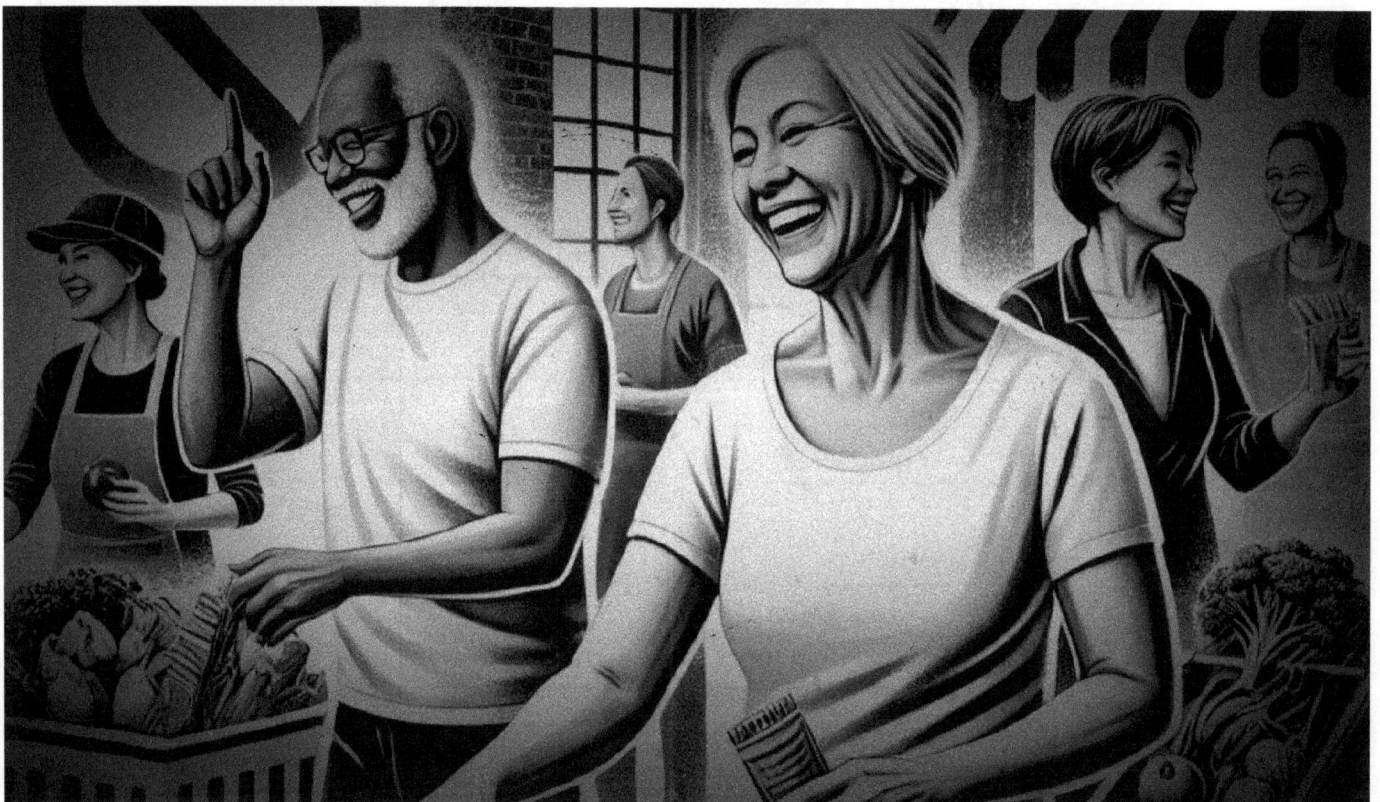

From Challenge to Change:
Real Participant Experiences

Real transformation happens when we take small, consistent steps toward better health. Each month, we challenge ourselves to build new habits, embrace positive changes, and support one another on this journey. But don't just take our word for it—hear from someone who has experienced the benefits firsthand. This testimonial highlights the real impact of this challenge and how it has helped others improve their well-being.

"As a busy nurse and self-confessed junk food junkie, I used to rely on chips, pretzels, and candy to get me through my hectic days. Junk food felt quick and convenient, but it left me feeling sluggish and always craving more. I even started hiding my snacks from my husband to avoid his judgment.

That's when I decided to try Dr. Fitness' 30-Day No Junk Food Challenge, and it completely transformed my habits and health. The challenge wasn't about deprivation—it helped me reset my taste buds and break free from unhealthy habits. By the end of the 30 days, I had replaced my chip-and-pretzel cravings with healthier snacks and organic protein options that suited my busy schedule. I'm now more energized, feel lighter, and have lost inches from my waist!

People constantly ask me how I achieved these changes, and they're always shocked when I say it's just from reducing junk food. I wholeheartedly recommend the No Junk Food Challenge to anyone who wants to feel amazing, improve their health, and take back control of what they eat."

— Linda, Nurse

Ditching Junk Food: How Eliminating Processed Snacks Transforms Your Health

From chips and cookies to candy and fried foods, junk food is designed to be addictive. While it might be tasty and convenient, these highly processed foods often leave us feeling sluggish, bloated, and craving more. The No Junk Food Challenge isn't about deprivation—it's about breaking free from unhealthy habits, resetting your taste buds, and discovering how amazing you can feel when you nourish your body with real food.

1. Breaking the Cycle of Food Addiction
Junk food is carefully engineered to make you crave more, combining sugar, salt, and unhealthy fats to trigger reward centers in your brain. By eliminating these foods for a month, you give your body a chance to reset, reducing cravings and making it easier to enjoy natural, whole foods.

2. Improved Digestion and Less Bloating
Processed junk food is often loaded with artificial ingredients, preservatives, and low-quality oils that can wreak havoc on your digestive system. Removing these foods allows your gut to heal, leading to reduced bloating, more regular digestion, and better absorption of essential nutrients.

3. More Stable Energy and Fewer Crashes
Junk food tends to be high in refined sugars and simple carbohydrates, which spike blood sugar levels and lead to inevitable crashes. Without these energy dips, you'll experience more consistent energy throughout the day, avoiding the afternoon slump and brain fog that come with processed snacks.

4. Natural Weight Regulation
Junk food is calorie-dense but nutrient-poor, meaning it's easy to overeat without feeling satisfied. By switching to whole foods, your body naturally regulates hunger and satiety, making it easier to maintain a healthy weight without counting calories or feeling deprived.

5. Reduced Inflammation and Clearer Skin
Highly processed foods contribute to inflammation, which can manifest as joint pain, digestive issues, and even acne. Many people who eliminate junk food report clearer skin, reduced redness, and a more balanced complexion, thanks to fewer inflammatory triggers.

6. Better Mood and Mental Clarity
The artificial additives and excess sugar in junk food don't just affect your body—they also impact your mood and brain function. Studies show that diets high in processed foods are linked to increased anxiety and depression. By eating whole, nutrient-dense foods, you can support brain health, stabilize mood, and improve mental clarity.

7. Discovering the Joy of Real Food
When you remove processed junk from your diet, your taste buds begin to change. You start appreciating the natural sweetness of fruit, the richness of fresh vegetables, and the satisfying flavors of homemade meals. This challenge encourages you to explore new, healthy snacks and meals that leave you feeling full, energized, and nourished.

Final Thoughts: A Lifestyle Shift, Not a Diet
The No Junk Food Challenge is about making mindful choices, not about perfection. By the end of 30 days, you'll likely feel lighter, more energetic, and in control of your eating habits. Whether you decide to cut out junk food entirely or simply reduce it in the future, this challenge sets the foundation for a healthier, more balanced lifestyle.

Are you ready to break free from processed foods and fuel your body with real nourishment? Your future self will thank you!

SMART *Goals*

Write your overall goal for this month's challenge.
- **S**pecific: What exactly will you do?
- **M**easurable: How will you track your progress?
- **A**chievable: How can you realistically achieve this goal?
- **R**elevant: Why does this goal matter to you?
- **T**ime-Bound: What is the timeframe?

_____

_____

_____

_____

_____

_____

_____

_____

_____

_____

_____

June marks the start of summer, making it an ideal time to clean up your diet and focus on nourishing your body. The 30-Day No Junk Food Challenge encourages you to eliminate processed and unhealthy foods, replacing them with wholesome, nutrient-dense options that leave you feeling energized and refreshed.

Fuel Your Body with
Nutrient-Rich Foods

Why Take the No Junk Food Challenge?

Cutting out junk food can lead to noticeable improvements in your health and well-being, including:

- Increased energy levels and stamina.
- Better digestion and reduced bloating.
- Clearer skin and a healthier complexion.
- Enhanced mental clarity and focus.
- Reduced risk of chronic health conditions like obesity and diabetes.

Tips for Success

1. Identify Your Triggers: Recognize the situations or emotions that lead you to reach for junk food and plan healthier alternatives.
2. Stock Your Pantry Wisely: Replace chips, cookies, and sugary snacks with nuts, seeds, fresh fruit, and whole-grain crackers.
3. Meal Prep: Prepare healthy meals and snacks in advance to avoid the temptation of fast or processed foods.
4. Hydrate: Sometimes thirst can be mistaken for hunger. Drink plenty of water throughout the day.

Common Pitfalls and How to Overcome Them

- Cravings: Satisfy sweet cravings with natural options like fresh berries or a piece of dark chocolate.
- Convenience Overload: Keep easy-to-grab healthy snacks on hand for busy days.
- Social Pressure: Be prepared with a response when offered junk food at events, such as, "I'm trying something new and focusing on healthier options this month."

Sample Daily Action Plan

- Morning: Enjoy a nutrient-packed smoothie made with spinach, frozen berries, and almond milk.
- Afternoon: Snack on raw veggies with hummus or a handful of mixed nuts.
- Evening: Prepare a balanced dinner with lean protein, whole grains, and roasted vegetables.
- Snack: Savor a slice of avocado toast or a small bowl of air-popped popcorn.

By the end of June, you'll notice a transformation in how you feel and fuel your body. This challenge is a powerful step toward creating healthier eating habits that last a lifetime.

June

- Junk food isn't just about taste—it's a habit. Breaking the cycle helps you regain control over your cravings.
- Real food gives you real energy. Processed snacks lead to crashes, while whole foods provide steady fuel.
- Your taste buds will adjust. The less junk you eat, the better natural foods will taste.
- You're feeding your future self. Every good choice supports better digestion, weight, and mental clarity.

Encouragement & Mindset Shift

Junk food is designed to be addictive, but you're stronger than your cravings. This challenge helps you reset your body, improve energy levels, and take control of your eating habits.

- Cravings Mean You're Breaking the Cycle – The first week may be tough, but every time you resist, your brain rewires itself to crave healthier options.
- You'll Notice More Energy – Processed foods cause energy crashes, while whole foods give your body steady fuel.
- Your Taste Buds Will Reset – After a few weeks, naturally sweet foods will taste better, and junk food won't seem as appealing.
- This Isn't About Perfection—It's About Progress – If you slip up, don't quit. Get back on track with the next meal.
- You're Gaining, Not Losing – By cutting out junk, you're gaining better digestion, clearer skin, fewer cravings, and long-term health benefits.

By the end of this challenge, you'll crave less junk, enjoy whole foods more, and feel in control of your food choices.

Looking for Junk Food Alternatives?

Try These Instead!

Craving junk food doesn't mean you have to give up flavor, crunch, or satisfaction—it just means making smarter choices that nourish your body instead of depleting it. Use these swaps to satisfy your cravings while staying committed to the challenge.

If You Crave... Try This Instead!

Chips & Salty Snacks... Crunchy & Satisfying Alternatives
- Air-popped popcorn with olive oil and sea salt instead of buttered or flavored popcorn.
- Roasted chickpeas, edamame, or nuts for a crunchy, protein-packed snack.
- Sliced cucumbers, bell peppers, or celery with hummus for a fresh, crisp bite.
- Baked or air-fried sweet potato fries instead of greasy fast-food fries.

Candy & Sugary Treats... Naturally Sweet & Guilt-Free Options
- Dark chocolate (70%+ cacao) instead of milk chocolate or candy bars.
- Frozen grapes, banana slices, or mango chunks for a refreshing treat.
- Medjool dates stuffed with almond butter for a chewy, sweet fix.
- Homemade energy bites made with oats, nut butter, and honey.

Fast Food & Processed Meals... Healthy, Quick Alternatives
- A homemade grain bowl with brown rice, veggies, and lean protein instead of takeout.
- A whole wheat wrap with avocado, turkey, and greens instead of a drive-thru sandwich.
- Baked salmon or grilled chicken with roasted vegetables instead of fried foods.
- A simple smoothie with protein, fruit, and almond milk instead of a sugary shake.

Sugary Drinks & Soda... Refreshing & Natural Choices
- Infused water with citrus, cucumber, or berries for a flavorful alternative.
- Herbal iced tea with mint or lemon instead of sweetened bottled teas.
- Sparkling water with a splash of 100% fruit juice instead of soda.
- Coconut water for natural hydration instead of energy drinks.

Ice Cream & Dairy-Based Desserts... Creamy, Healthy Replacements
- Frozen blended bananas ("nice cream") with cacao powder for a creamy treat.
- Greek yogurt with honey and fruit instead of sugary flavored yogurts.
- Chia pudding with almond milk and cinnamon instead of store-bought puddings.
- Coconut or almond milk ice cream instead of dairy-based options.

Pastries & Baked Goods... Wholesome, Satisfying Options
- Oatmeal with cinnamon and nuts instead of sugary cereal.
- Whole grain toast with almond butter instead of pastries.
- Protein pancakes made with banana, oats, and eggs instead of processed mixes.
- Homemade muffins with whole wheat flour and natural sweeteners instead of store-bought muffins.

Journaling Prompts
JUNE

1 What cravings have been the hardest to resist, and how have you managed them?

_____

_____

_____

_____

2 How does eating whole, unprocessed foods make you feel compared to junk food?

_____

_____

_____

_____

3 What new healthy snacks or meals have you discovered during this challenge?

_____

_____

_____

_____

Craving Control: Your 30-Day Junk-Free Tracker

This challenge helps you build awareness around cravings while focusing on nourishing, whole foods. Each day, log any junk food cravings, note what triggered them, and track how you managed to overcome them. Use the space provided to list the healthy foods you ate and reflect on how they made you feel. By the end of 30 days, you'll have a better understanding of your eating habits, improved self-control, and a foundation for making healthier choices long-term!

Feel free to copy this page to track additional weeks and continue your progress.

Date	Craving (What Food)?	What Triggered It?	How Did I Overcome It?	Healthy Foods I Ate Today	Notes (Energy, Mood, Hunger Levels)
6/1	Chips	Boredom	Ate almonds instead	Grilled salmon, quinoa, veggies	Less bloated than usual

July

Drink A Gallon Water Challenge

Stay hydrated and thrive. This chapter explains the role of water in weight loss, mental clarity, and overall health. Includes practical advice for reaching your daily water intake goal.

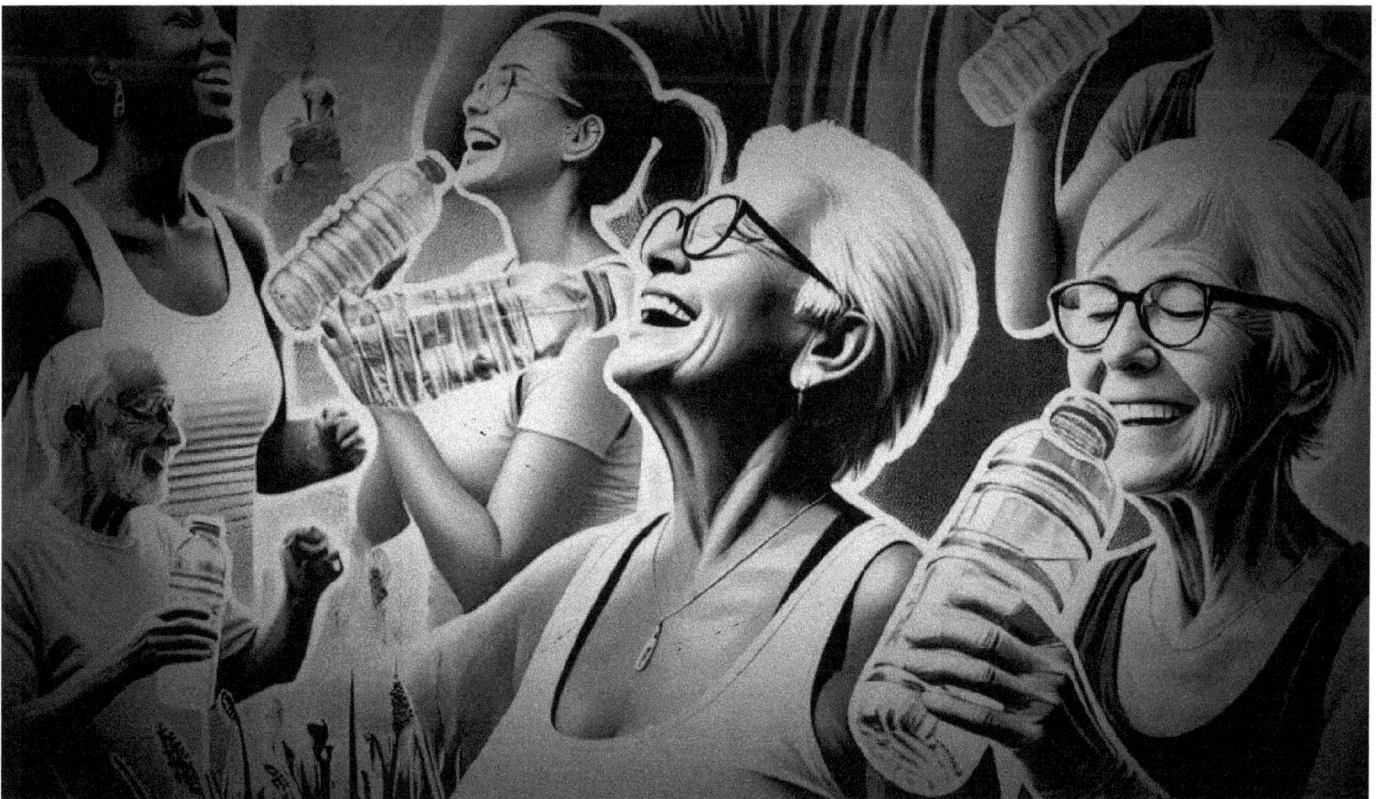

From Challenge to Change:
Real Participant Experiences

Real transformation happens when we take small, consistent steps toward better health. Each month, we challenge ourselves to build new habits, embrace positive changes, and support one another on this journey. But don't just take our word for it—hear from someone who has experienced the benefits firsthand. This testimonial highlights the real impact of this challenge and how it has helped others improve their well-being.

"I'm a 65-year-old retired grandma, and I was looking forward to spending more quality time with my grandchildren. But I felt constantly drained—headaches, fatigue, and no energy to keep up with them. My doctor couldn't find anything wrong, so I assumed it was just part of aging.

That's when my daughter suggested I try the 30-Day Drink a Gallon of Water a Day Challenge after hearing Dr. Fitness on the radio. At first, I thought, 'I already drink water every day; how hard can it be?' But drinking a full gallon was a completely different experience. I realized I'd been sipping here and there, which wasn't enough to stay hydrated.

By committing to this challenge, everything changed. My energy came back, my headaches disappeared, and the brain fog lifted. It felt incredible to finally feel like myself again! I learned how vital proper hydration is and how easily we undervalue something so simple. I'm so grateful to this challenge—it's given me my energy back and helped me keep up with my grandkids!"

Monica - grandma

The Power of Hydration: How Drinking a Gallon of Water a Day Transforms Your Health

Water is the foundation of life, yet many of us don't drink nearly enough of it. Dehydration can sneak up in subtle ways—fatigue, headaches, brain fog, dry skin, and even sugar cravings. The Drink a Gallon of Water a Day Hydration Challenge is designed to help you experience the incredible benefits of proper hydration firsthand. By making water a priority for 30 days, you'll likely see improvements in your energy, digestion, skin, and overall well-being.

1. More Energy and Less Fatigue
Even mild dehydration can lead to low energy levels, sluggishness, and difficulty concentrating. When your body doesn't have enough water, it has to work harder to circulate oxygen and nutrients. Drinking a gallon a day keeps your cells hydrated, helping you feel more alert, focused, and energized throughout the day.

2. Supports Digestion and Prevents Bloating
Water plays a crucial role in digestion, helping break down food and move it through the digestive tract. Without enough hydration, the body struggles to properly digest meals, leading to bloating, constipation, and discomfort. Drinking plenty of water ensures smooth digestion and nutrient absorption.

3. Clears Up Skin and Enhances Radiance
Skin is the body's largest organ, and dehydration often shows up in the form of dryness, dullness, and breakouts. Proper hydration flushes out toxins, improves elasticity, and helps reduce the appearance of fine lines and acne. Many people notice a visible glow within just a few weeks of drinking more water.

4. Reduces Cravings and Supports Weight Management
Thirst is often mistaken for hunger, leading to unnecessary snacking and cravings for sugar or salty foods. Staying hydrated helps regulate appetite, reducing unnecessary food intake. Plus, water helps the body metabolize fat more efficiently, making it easier to maintain a healthy weight.

5. Improves Joint Health and Reduces Inflammation
Water acts as a natural lubricant for joints, reducing stiffness and discomfort. When the body is well-hydrated, it experiences less inflammation, which can lead to decreased joint pain and greater mobility—especially beneficial for those with arthritis or an active lifestyle.

6. Detoxifies the Body and Improves Kidney Function
The kidneys rely on water to filter toxins and waste products from the bloodstream. When properly hydrated, your body eliminates waste more efficiently through urine and sweat, reducing the risk of kidney stones and improving overall organ function.

7. Strengthens Mental Clarity and Focus
The brain is made up of about 75% water, and even slight dehydration can impair memory, focus, and mood. Drinking a gallon a day helps keep cognitive function sharp, improving productivity and reducing the likelihood of mental fatigue.

Final Thoughts: The Key to Long-Term Health
The Hydration Challenge isn't just about drinking more water for a month—it's about experiencing the long-term benefits of staying properly hydrated. Once you see how much better you feel, you'll be more mindful of making hydration a daily priority. Whether you continue drinking a gallon a day or simply increase your intake, this challenge teaches you how water is one of the simplest yet most powerful ways to support overall health.

Are you ready to see what a difference hydration can make? Your body is craving it—drink up!

SMART *Goals*

Write your overall goal for this month's challenge.
- **S**pecific: What exactly will you do?
- **M**easurable: How will you track your progress?
- **A**chievable: How can you realistically achieve this goal?
- **R**elevant: Why does this goal matter to you?
- **T**ime-Bound: What is the timeframe?

_____

_____

_____

_____

_____

_____

_____

_____

_____

_____

_____

_____

July's heat makes it an ideal time to focus on hydration. The 30-Day Drink-A-Gallon Water Challenge encourages you to drink a gallon of water daily to optimize your body's functions, improve energy levels, and enhance overall well-being.

Hydrate for Energy, Health and Clarity

Why Take the Drink-A-Gallon Water Challenge?

Proper hydration is essential for nearly every bodily function. Drinking a gallon of water daily can:

- Improve energy levels and reduce fatigue.
- Promote clear, glowing skin by flushing out toxins.
- Enhance digestion and support weight loss.
- Prevent headaches caused by dehydration.
- Boost overall mood and mental clarity.

Tips for Success

1. Invest in a Gallon Jug: A reusable gallon-sized water bottle makes tracking intake easier.
2. Break It Down: Drink in increments throughout the day (e.g., 16 ounces every hour).
3. Add Flavor: Infuse water with fruits, herbs, or cucumber for variety.
4. Pair It With Meals: Drink a glass before and during meals to stay on track.

Common Pitfalls and How to Overcome Them

- Forgetting to Drink: Set reminders on your phone or use a water-tracking app.
- Overwhelmed by the Amount: Start with smaller goals, such as half a gallon, and work up.
- Bathroom Breaks: Your body will adjust to increased hydration within a few days.

Sample Daily Action Plan

- Morning: Drink 16 ounces of water upon waking.
- Afternoon: Carry a water bottle with you and sip consistently throughout the day.
- Evening: Finish the last portion of your gallon by dinnertime to avoid late-night trips to the bathroom.

By the end of July, you'll feel the remarkable difference proper hydration makes in your energy, mood, and overall health.

July

- Water is the easiest way to boost health. Better hydration leads to more energy, clearer skin, and improved digestion.
- Your body thrives when it's hydrated. Joint pain, fatigue, and cravings all improve when you drink enough water.
- If you feel sluggish, drink water first. Dehydration often feels like hunger, tiredness, or brain fog.
- Hydration is a habit. The more you drink water, the more your body will crave it naturally.

Encouragement & Mindset Shift

Water is the foundation of energy, mental clarity, digestion, and overall health. Most people don't drink enough, but once you start prioritizing hydration, you'll feel the difference almost immediately. This challenge isn't just about drinking more water—it's about learning to listen to your body and giving it what it truly needs.

- Water is the easiest way to improve your health. It helps with digestion, energy, skin, and mental clarity.
- You're Rebuilding a Hydration Habit – If you're not used to drinking this much water, your body will adjust, and you'll start craving it naturally.
- Dehydration Feels Like Hunger & Fatigue – Before reaching for a snack, drink water first and see how you feel.
- Track Your Wins – Notice improvements in skin, digestion, and energy. Even minor changes will keep you motivated.
- Make It Enjoyable – Try infused water, herbal teas, or sparkling water to keep things interesting.

By the end of this challenge, drinking water will feel effortless, and your body will thrive from proper hydration!

Looking for Hydration Alternatives?

Try These Instead!

Drinking a gallon of water each day may seem challenging, but staying hydrated doesn't have to be boring! If you struggle to drink enough water, try these flavorful, refreshing, and creative alternatives to make your hydration habit easier and more enjoyable.

If You Crave… Try This Instead!

Plain Water Feels Boring… Naturally Flavored Water
- Infused water with cucumber, lemon, lime, or mint for a refreshing taste.
- Berry-infused water with strawberries, raspberries, or blueberries for a subtle sweetness.
- Herbal tea (iced or hot) with chamomile, hibiscus, or peppermint for variety.
- Water with a splash of fresh citrus juice (lemon, lime, or orange) for a little zing.

You Need a Hydration Boost… Natural Electrolyte Drinks
- Coconut water for hydration and electrolyte balance without artificial additives.
- Watermelon juice blended with a pinch of sea salt for natural replenishment.
- Homemade electrolyte water with water, lemon juice, a pinch of salt, and honey.
- Cucumber and celery juice for a hydrating, mineral-rich option.

Craving Bubbles… Fizzy & Sparkling Alternatives
- Sparkling water with a splash of fruit juice for a soda-like experience.
- Carbonated mineral water with lime or cucumber for a crisp, refreshing drink.
- Kombucha (low-sugar) for a probiotic-rich, tangy alternative.
- Club soda with a squeeze of grapefruit or pomegranate juice.

You Forget to Drink Water… Hydration Hacks
- Keep a large reusable water bottle with you at all times.
- Set a reminder alarm every hour to take a few sips.
- Use a water-tracking app or mark your bottle with hourly goals.
- Drink a full glass of water before each meal as a habit trigger.

You Prefer Sweet Drinks… Naturally Sweet Hydration
- Cold hibiscus or berry herbal tea with a touch of honey.
- Coconut water with a dash of vanilla or cinnamon for a subtle sweetness.
- Aloe vera juice mixed with water for a soothing, mildly sweet drink.
- Chia seed water with lemon and honey for hydration plus fiber.

You Need a Cooling Drink… Ice-Cold Hydration Ideas
- Freeze fruit into ice cubes to add flavor as they melt.
- Make homemade fruit ice pops with blended fruit and water.
- Blend coconut water with frozen mango or pineapple for a slushy treat.
- Keep a pitcher of cold infused water in the fridge for easy access.

Journaling Prompts
JULY

1 How does drinking a gallon of water each day affect your energy, mood, and skin?

_____

_____

_____

_____

2 What creative ways have you used to stay hydrated (e.g., flavored water, reusable bottles)?

_____

_____

_____

_____

3 How does proper hydration influence your cravings or appetite?

_____

_____

_____

_____

Stay Hydrated: Your 30-Day Water Log

Staying hydrated is key to better energy, digestion, skin health, and overall well-being! Use this tracker to monitor your daily intake by shading in the water bottle as you drink throughout the day. Each section represents 16 ounces, and your goal is to fill all eight sections by the end of the day. Check in with yourself by rating how you feel and reflecting on any changes. By the end of the 30 days, you'll be amazed at how much proper hydration impacts your body and mind!

Feel free to copy this page to track additional weeks and continue your progress.

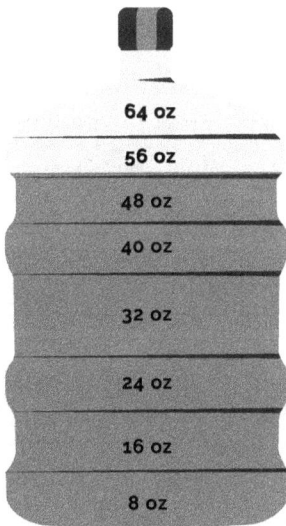

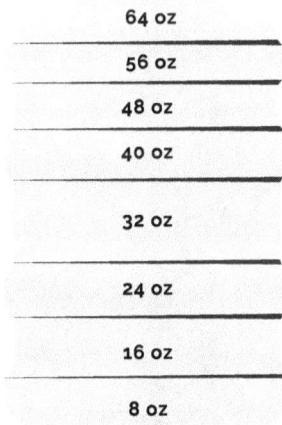

Monday

| 64 oz |
| 56 oz |
| 48 oz |
| 40 oz |
| 32 oz |
| 24 oz |
| 16 oz |
| 8 oz |

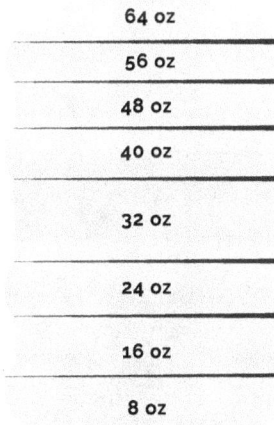

Tuesday

| 64 oz |
| 56 oz |
| 48 oz |
| 40 oz |
| 32 oz |
| 24 oz |
| 16 oz |
| 8 oz |

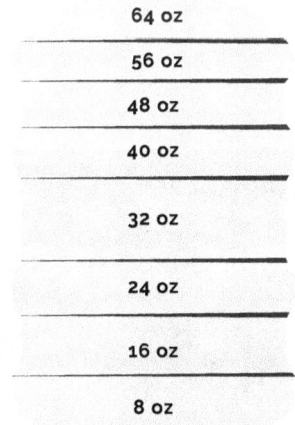

Wednesday

| 64 oz |
| 56 oz |
| 48 oz |
| 40 oz |
| 32 oz |
| 24 oz |
| 16 oz |
| 8 oz |

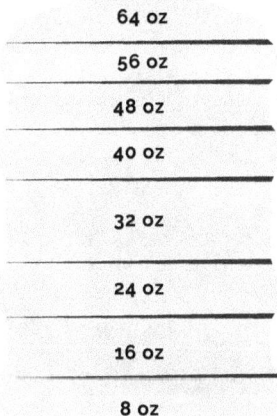

Thursday

| 64 oz |
| 56 oz |
| 48 oz |
| 40 oz |
| 32 oz |
| 24 oz |
| 16 oz |
| 8 oz |

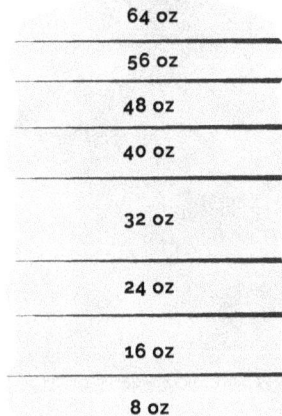

Friday

| 64 oz |
| 56 oz |
| 48 oz |
| 40 oz |
| 32 oz |
| 24 oz |
| 16 oz |
| 8 oz |

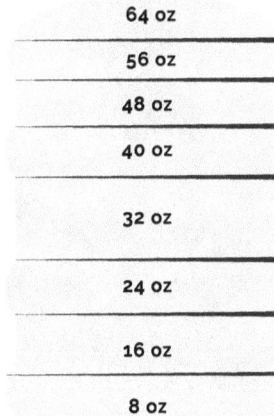

Saturday

| 64 oz |
| 56 oz |
| 48 oz |
| 40 oz |
| 32 oz |
| 24 oz |
| 16 oz |
| 8 oz |

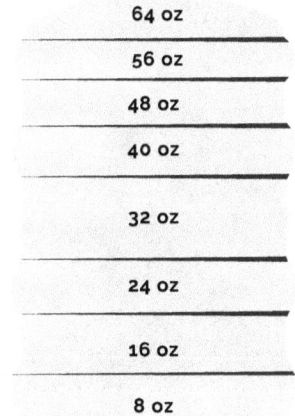

Sunday

| 64 oz |
| 56 oz |
| 48 oz |
| 40 oz |
| 32 oz |
| 24 oz |
| 16 oz |
| 8 oz |

August

No Nicotine Challenge

Take a step toward freedom by cutting out nicotine. With tips for managing cravings, using substitutes like the patch, and building a support system, this chapter provides the foundation for a healthier lifestyle.

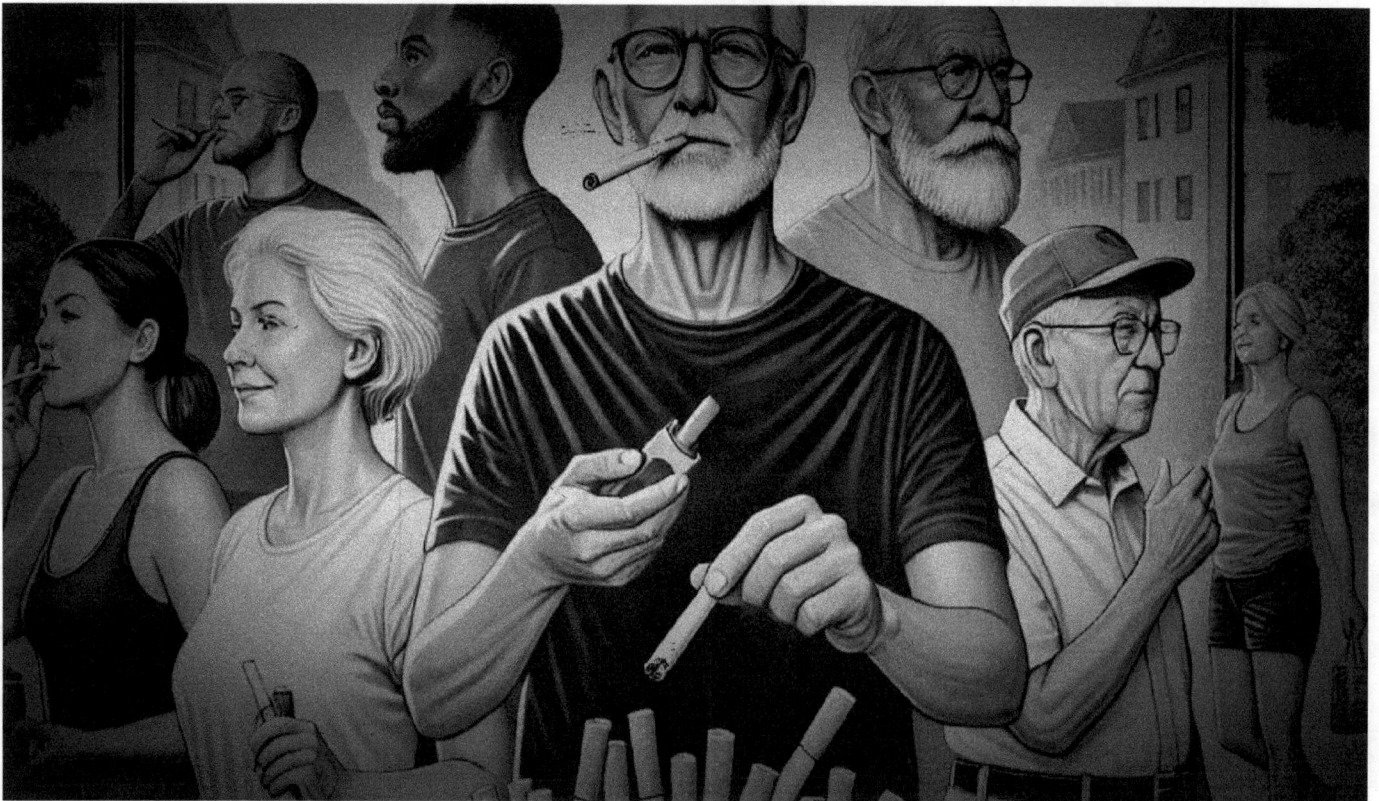

From Challenge to Change:
Real Participant Experiences

Real transformation happens when we take small, consistent steps toward better health. Each month, we challenge ourselves to build new habits, embrace positive changes, and support one another on this journey. But don't just take our word for it—hear from someone who has experienced the benefits firsthand. This testimonial highlights the real impact of this challenge and how it has helped others improve their well-being.

"I smoked for 30 years and always believed I wasn't truly addicted to cigarettes—I thought I could stop anytime I wanted. When I took the challenge to quit for just 30 days, I was sure it would be easy. Imagine my surprise when I found myself failing again and again, at least once a week. Each time I lit up, I felt defeated. But what made all the difference was the support I received from Dr. Fitness. Every time I reached out, feeling frustrated, his response never wavered: "What did you learn from the fail? And just because you failed doesn't mean you should quit trying."

That simple, steadfast encouragement kept me motivated. With each failure, I discovered hidden triggers and learned to work through them. My original goal was only to prove I wasn't addicted, but after six months of trying again and again, I finally conquered the challenge—30 nicotine-free days. At that point, I realized I didn't need nicotine anymore. That's when I made the decision to quit smoking for good. Go figure, right?

The challenge not only helped me beat nicotine but also drastically improved my health. My lungs and stamina got stronger. I could take deeper breaths, and my physical endurance improved dramatically. Plus, knowing I'd reduced my risk of heart disease? That was a true win for my long-term health.

This challenge was more than just a test of willpower—it was a chance to reclaim my life. If you're considering kicking nicotine, the 30-Day No Nicotine Challenge is the best place to start. You might just surprise yourself—like I did."

—Carl, Nicotine-Free Now

Breaking Free from Nicotine: How a Month Without It Can Change Your Life

Nicotine is one of the most addictive substances in the world, keeping millions of people hooked on cigarettes, vaping, and other tobacco products. While quitting can feel overwhelming, the benefits of a nicotine-free life begin almost immediately. The No Nicotine Challenge is an opportunity to reclaim your health, regain control over cravings, and experience what life feels like without dependency. By committing to 30 days nicotine-free, you'll set yourself up for long-term success and greater well-being.

1. Immediate Health Improvements
Just 20 minutes after your last nicotine use, your heart rate and blood pressure start to normalize. Within 12 hours, carbon monoxide levels in your blood drop, allowing oxygen to circulate more efficiently. After a few days, lung function begins to improve, making breathing easier and increasing energy levels.

2. Restoring Brain Chemistry and Mental Clarity
Nicotine hijacks the brain's reward system, creating cycles of cravings and withdrawals. When you quit, your dopamine levels begin to rebalance, leading to improved mood, better focus, and more emotional stability. While the first few days may feel challenging, many people report increased mental clarity and a greater sense of calm after the initial withdrawal phase.

3. Strengthening Your Lungs and Circulatory System
Nicotine and tobacco weaken lung function, reducing oxygen intake and making physical activity harder. Within a few weeks of quitting, lung capacity begins to increase, allowing for deeper breaths, improved endurance, and a stronger heart. Your risk of heart disease also drops significantly.

4. Improved Sleep and Reduced Fatigue
Nicotine disrupts sleep patterns by stimulating the nervous system, making it harder to fall and stay asleep. Once you quit, your body can enter deeper, more restorative sleep cycles, leading to better energy levels, improved concentration, and reduced feelings of exhaustion.

5. Financial Savings and Increased Freedom
Smoking and vaping are expensive habits that add up over time. The average smoker spends thousands of dollars a year on cigarettes or nicotine products. By quitting, you not only save money, but you also gain the freedom to enjoy life without constantly thinking about your next nicotine fix.

6. Better Skin, Hair, and Overall Appearance
Nicotine restricts blood flow, depriving skin and hair of essential nutrients. This can lead to premature aging, dull complexion, and hair thinning. Quitting nicotine restores proper circulation, helping skin regain its natural glow and hair become healthier and stronger.

7. Breaking the Habit for Good
Quitting nicotine isn't just about physical addiction—it's about changing routines and behaviors associated with it. Whether you smoke during stress, after meals, or with coffee, this challenge encourages you to find healthier alternatives. By the end of 30 days, many people feel empowered to continue their nicotine-free journey long-term.

Final Thoughts: A New Beginning
The No Nicotine Challenge is a powerful step toward a healthier, longer, and more vibrant life. While the first few days may feel difficult, every day without nicotine is a victory. By the end of this challenge, you'll have a new perspective on your body's strength and resilience—and you may just find that you never want to go back.

Are you ready to break free and take control of your health? Your future self will thank you for every day you stay nicotine-free.

SMART *Goals*

Write your overall goal for this month's challenge.
- **S**pecific: What exactly will you do?
- **M**easurable: How will you track your progress?
- **A**chievable: How can you realistically achieve this goal?
- **R**elevant: Why does this goal matter to you?
- **T**ime-Bound: What is the timeframe?

_____

_____

_____

_____

_____

_____

_____

_____

_____

_____

_____

_____

August offers a fresh start with the 30-Day No Nicotine Challenge. Whether you smoke or use other forms of nicotine, this challenge empowers you to quit and embrace a healthier, more vibrant life.

Break Free and
Breathe Easy

Why Take the No Nicotine Challenge?

Quitting nicotine is one of the best decisions you can make for your health. Benefits include:

- Improved lung capacity and breathing.
- Reduced risk of heart disease and cancer.
- Enhanced sense of taste and smell.
- Increased energy and improved sleep quality.
- Freedom from dependency and cost savings.

Tips for Success

1. Identify Triggers: Recognize situations that lead to nicotine use and plan distractions or alternatives.
2. Find Support: Join a support group or talk to friends and family for encouragement.
3. Use Replacements: Chew gum, use nicotine patches, or practice deep breathing to ease cravings.
4. Track Progress: Celebrate milestones (1 day, 1 week, 1 month) to stay motivated.

Common Pitfalls and How to Overcome Them

- Intense Cravings: Distract yourself with physical activity, hobbies, or meditation.
- Stress Triggers: Use stress-relief techniques like yoga or journaling.
- Slip-Ups: Don't give up. Reflect on what led to the slip and recommit to the challenge.

Sample Daily Action Plan

- Morning: Reflect on your reasons for quitting and set your intention for the day.
- Afternoon: Keep sugar-free gum or a healthy snack on hand for cravings.
- Evening: Journal about your progress and the positive changes you're noticing.

By the end of August, you'll feel proud of your progress and motivated to continue living nicotine-free. Let this challenge be the first step toward a healthier future.

August

- Cravings don't last—resistance makes them weaker. If you wait 10 minutes, most urges will pass.
- You're breaking the cycle, not just quitting nicotine. This challenge is about freedom from addiction.
- Every cigarette you skip is a victory. Each day without nicotine lowers your risk of disease and strengthens your lungs.
- You are in control. Nicotine doesn't own you—you're proving to yourself that you're stronger.

Encouragement & Mindset Shift

Quitting nicotine is one of the best things you can do for your health, but it takes commitment and patience. This challenge isn't just about quitting a habit—it's about gaining back control, breathing easier, and feeling better every day.

- Cravings Are Temporary, Freedom Is Permanent – Each craving lasts only a few minutes. Distract yourself, take a deep breath, or drink water. Every time you resist, you're one step closer to breaking free.
- Your Body Starts Healing Immediately – In just 24 hours, your risk of heart disease drops. Within weeks, your lungs start to repair, and your energy improves.
- This Is About Strength, Not Willpower – You're not losing anything by quitting—you're gaining better health, more money, and a longer life.
- Break the Habit Loop – If you smoke out of stress, replace that action with breathing exercises, stretching, or chewing gum.
- Every Smoke-Free Day Is a Win – Focus on the victories, not the cravings. You're proving to yourself that you're stronger than nicotine.

By the end of this challenge, you'll feel empowered, breathe easier, and know that nicotine no longer controls you.

Looking for Nicotine Alternatives?

Try These Instead!

Quitting nicotine is one of the most powerful choices you can make for your health, but breaking the habit can be tough. Whether you smoke, vape, or use other nicotine products, having a plan and healthy alternatives will help you manage cravings and stay committed. Try these proven swaps to help you through the challenge.

If You Crave… Try This Instead!
The Oral Fixation… Keep Your Mouth Busy
- Sugar-free gum or mints to satisfy the need for chewing.
- Crunchy snacks like carrot sticks, celery, or nuts for a satisfying bite.
- A straw or cinnamon stick to mimic the hand-to-mouth motion of smoking.
- Herbal tea or flavored water to keep your mouth occupied.

The Hand Habit… Keep Your Hands Engaged
- A fidget toy, stress ball, or pen to keep your hands busy.
- Holding a cup of tea, water, or another healthy beverage.
- Playing with a coin, keychain, or piece of jewelry in your pocket.
- Knitting, doodling, or playing a game on your phone when cravings hit.

The Nicotine Rush… Find a Healthy Energy Boost
- A quick walk or stretching to re-energize naturally.
- Deep breathing exercises to release tension and refocus.
- Drinking a glass of cold water to refresh and reset.
- Eating a high-protein snack to stabilize energy levels.

The Stress Reliever… Manage Stress in a New Way
- Deep breathing or meditation to calm the mind.
- Journaling to track emotions and triggers.
- Listening to music, a podcast, or nature sounds for relaxation.
- Calling a supportive friend instead of reaching for nicotine.

The After-Meal Urge… Replace the Habit with a New Routine
- Going for a short walk after eating instead of smoking.
- Drinking herbal tea or chewing gum after meals.
- Brushing your teeth right after eating to signal the end of the meal.
- Practicing mindful eating to enjoy and savor your food fully.

Social Triggers… Stay Engaged Without Nicotine
- Holding a non-alcoholic drink in social settings to keep your hands occupied.
- Letting close friends and family know about your challenge for extra support.
- Practicing a short mantra like "I'm choosing my health" when cravings hit.
- Removing yourself from tempting situations if needed.

Journaling Prompts
AUGUST

1 What are your biggest triggers for nicotine use, and how can you replace them with healthier habits?

_____

_____

_____

_____

2 How do you feel physically and emotionally after going a full day without nicotine?

_____

_____

_____

_____

3 What long-term benefits do you hope to gain by eliminating nicotine from your life?

_____

_____

_____

_____

Breaking Free: Daily Tracker for a Nicotine-Free Life

Quitting nicotine is one of the best decisions you can make for your health, and this tracker will help you stay on track. Each day, check off your nicotine-free progress, log any cravings, and note what triggered them. Use this space to reflect on the alternative actions you took to manage cravings and track how you're feeling along the way. By the end of 30 days, you'll see just how far you've come in reclaiming your health and freedom!

Feel free to copy this page to track additional weeks and continue your progress.

Date	Nicotine Free	When Did The Craving Hit?	What Triggered It?	Alternative Action Taken?	Notes (Mood, Energy, Progress)
8/1	✔	2:00 p.m.	Stress at work	Took deep breaths and drank water	Felt anxious but proud

September

Lose Belly Fat Challenge

Target your core and learn how to reduce visceral fat with focused nutrition and exercise. This chapter includes meal plans, workout suggestions, and advice for tracking progress without obsessing over numbers.

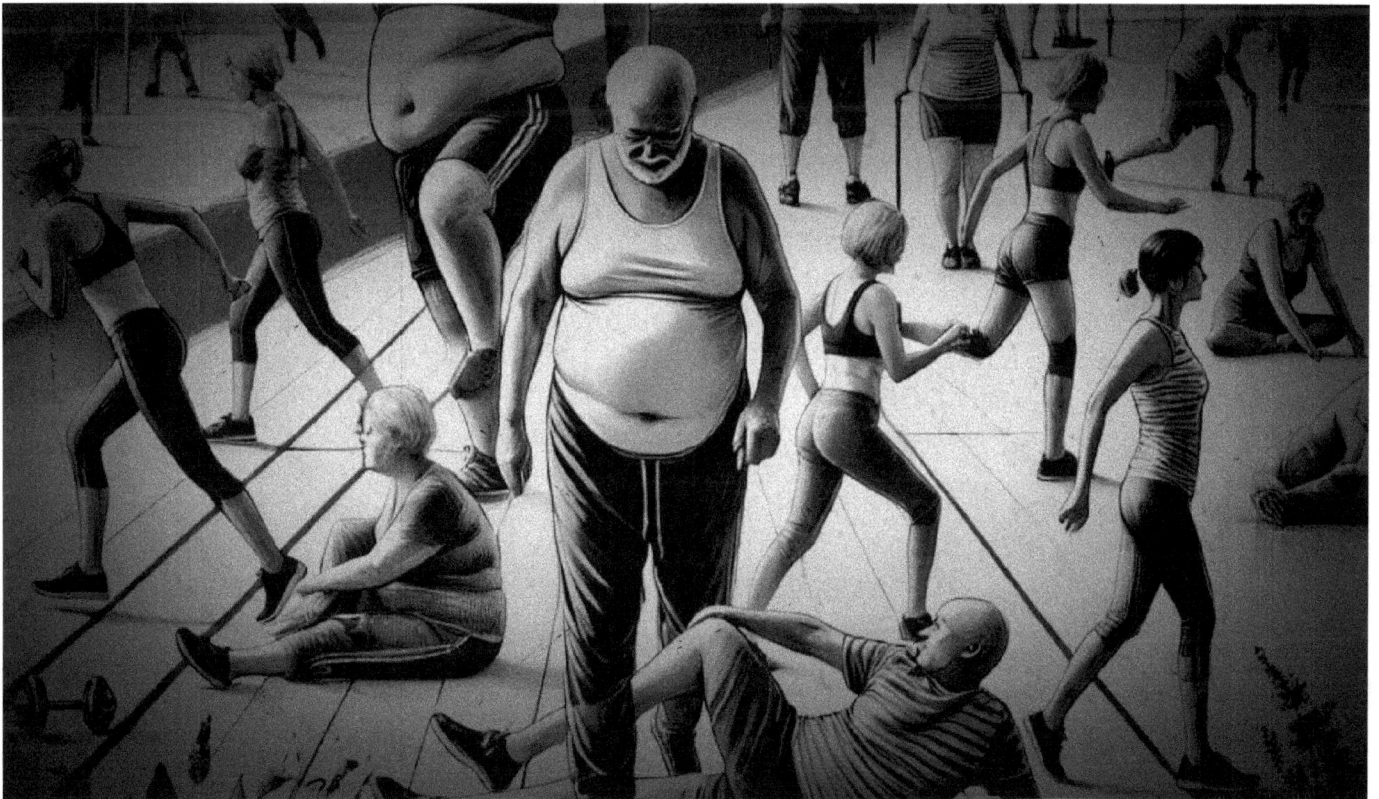

From Challenge to Change:
Real Participant Experiences

Real transformation happens when we take small, consistent steps toward better health. Each month, we challenge ourselves to build new habits, embrace positive changes, and support one another on this journey. But don't just take our word for it—hear from someone who has experienced the benefits firsthand. This testimonial highlights the real impact of this challenge and how it has helped others improve their well-being.

"Before joining the No Belly Fat Challenge, I never realized the true impact belly fat could have on my health. My family, including myself, always carried a little extra weight around the midsection, and it didn't seem like a big deal. My doctor never mentioned it, so I thought it was just part of life. But when I started struggling with high blood pressure, trouble sleeping, and pre-diabetes, I knew I needed to make a change.

One day, my husband and I were driving to lunch when we heard Dr. Fitness on the radio. He was talking about how belly fat isn't just about appearance—it's a serious health warning sign. Hearing him explain the connection between belly fat, diabetes, and high blood pressure hit close to home. When he mentioned the No Belly Fat Challenge, we decided to give it a shot.

The challenge completely transformed our lives. Over the course of the program, I lost 6 inches off my waist, and my husband lost 10 inches! Not only did we look better, but we felt incredible. We had more energy, experienced less stress, and even needed to reduce our blood pressure medications. The best part? My doctor confirmed I'm no longer pre-diabetic.

This wasn't a quick fix or a crash diet—it was about making sustainable changes to our nutrition and lifestyle. The mix of whole foods, effective workouts, and stress management techniques made the process feel achievable, even for two busy people like us.
I can't thank the No Belly Fat Challenge enough for giving my husband and me a fresh start. If you've been struggling with belly fat or early health warnings, don't hesitate—this program truly works!"

Rhonda- Accountant

Shedding Belly Fat: A 30-Day Challenge for a Healthier, Stronger You

Excess belly fat isn't just about appearance—it's closely linked to serious health risks, including heart disease, diabetes, and inflammation. The Lose Belly Fat Challenge is designed to help you break free from stubborn weight, boost your metabolism, and feel stronger from the inside out. This isn't about crash dieting—it's about sustainable changes that help your body burn fat efficiently while improving overall well-being.

1. Understanding Belly Fat: Why It's More Than Just Weight
There are two types of fat in the body: subcutaneous fat (just under the skin) and visceral fat (which surrounds organs). Visceral fat, particularly in the abdominal area, is the most dangerous because it releases inflammatory chemicals that increase the risk of chronic diseases. Reducing this type of fat improves both appearance and long-term health.

2. Prioritizing Whole Foods Over Processed Foods
The most effective way to lose belly fat is through nutrition. Cutting out processed foods, refined sugars, and unhealthy fats helps regulate blood sugar levels and reduce inflammation. Instead, focus on whole, nutrient-dense foods like lean proteins, vegetables, healthy fats, and fiber-rich carbohydrates to keep your metabolism active and prevent fat storage.

3. Strengthening the Core Beyond Crunches
While core exercises help tone abdominal muscles, they won't eliminate belly fat on their own. Instead, focus on full-body strength training and high-intensity interval training (HIIT) workouts. These workouts burn fat more efficiently by increasing muscle mass and improving metabolic function.

4. Managing Stress to Reduce Cortisol Levels
Chronic stress leads to high cortisol levels, which encourage fat storage—especially in the abdominal area. Incorporating stress-management techniques such as meditation, deep breathing, or even daily walks can help regulate cortisol and support fat loss.

5. Balancing Sleep for Fat-Burning Efficiency
Sleep is one of the most underrated tools for fat loss. Poor sleep disrupts hormone levels, leading to increased hunger and cravings. Aim for 7–9 hours of quality sleep per night to allow your body to recover, regulate metabolism, and support a healthy weight.

6. Staying Hydrated to Boost Metabolism
Drinking enough water helps flush toxins, improve digestion, and boost metabolism. Often, dehydration is mistaken for hunger, leading to unnecessary snacking. Drinking water before meals can help with portion control and keep your body functioning optimally.

7. Consistency Over Perfection
Losing belly fat isn't about following a restrictive diet for a few weeks—it's about developing habits that support long-term health. Small, consistent changes—like choosing whole foods, moving your body daily, and prioritizing sleep—lead to sustainable results.

Final Thoughts: A Stronger, Healthier You
The Lose Belly Fat Challenge isn't about unrealistic goals—it's about creating a lifestyle that helps you feel stronger, more energized, and more confident in your body. By the end of this challenge, you'll not only see changes in your waistline but also experience improvements in overall health, mental clarity, and physical strength.

Are you ready to take control of your health and feel your best? Your journey to a leaner, healthier you starts today!

SMART *Goals*

Write your overall goal for this month's challenge.
- **S**pecific: What exactly will you do?
- **M**easurable: How will you track your progress?
- **A**chievable: How can you realistically achieve this goal?
- **R**elevant: Why does this goal matter to you?
- **T**ime-Bound: What is the timeframe?

_____

_____

_____

_____

_____

_____

_____

_____

_____

_____

_____

_____

September is all about getting back to basics and focusing on your core health. The 30-Day Lose Belly Fat Challenge combines clean eating, targeted exercises, and mindfulness to reduce belly fat, enhance strength, and build confidence.

Target Your Core, Boost Confidence, And Build Strength

Why Take the Lose Belly Fat Challenge?

Belly fat isn't just about aesthetics; it's linked to significant health concerns. This challenge can:

- Reduce risks of heart disease and diabetes.
- Improve posture and core strength.
- Enhance energy levels and physical performance.
- Boost self-confidence with visible progress.

Tips for Success
1. Focus on Nutrition: Prioritize whole foods, lean proteins, and healthy fats while avoiding processed sugar and refined carbs.
2. Incorporate Cardio and Strength Training: Combine high-intensity interval training (HIIT) with core-targeting exercises like planks and Russian twists.
3. Stay Consistent: Set a schedule to ensure you stick to your workout and meal plans.
4. Hydrate: Proper hydration aids digestion and reduces bloating.

Common Pitfalls and How to Overcome Them
- Plateaus: Change up your exercise routine to keep your muscles challenged.
- Cravings: Use healthy snacks like nuts or fresh fruits to stay satisfied.
- Skipping Workouts: Prepare shorter, more intense sessions for busy days.

Sample Daily Action Plan
- Morning: Start with a 20-minute HIIT session focused on cardio and core.
- Afternoon: Enjoy a balanced lunch with lean protein, veggies, and healthy fats.
- Evening: End with a calming yoga stretch to release tension and strengthen your core.

By the end of September, you'll feel stronger, more energized, and more confident in your body. With a leaner core and healthier habits in place, you'll be empowered to continue your fitness journey and maintain lasting results.

September

- Core strength isn't just about looks—it's about health. A strong core helps with posture, digestion, and injury prevention.
- Every workout counts. Even 5-10 minutes of movement adds up over time.
- Food choices make the biggest impact. Processed foods store fat, but whole foods help your body burn it.
- This is about long-term wellness, not a quick fix. Consistency is more important than perfection.

Encouragement & Mindset Shift

Belly fat isn't just about appearance—it's about your health, energy, and long-term wellness. This challenge is about strengthening your core, eating smarter, and building lasting habits.

- Small Changes, Big Impact – It's not about extreme dieting. Daily movement, balanced meals, and consistency create lasting results.
- You Can't Spot-Reduce, But You Can Transform – Focusing on core exercises, strength training, and whole foods will reshape your body over time.
- This Isn't Just About Weight—It's About Energy – Less belly fat means better digestion, lower stress, and a stronger body.
- Every Workout Counts – Even 5-10 minutes of core exercises daily helps build strength and burn fat over time.
- Fuel, Don't Restrict – You're not starving yourself—you're fueling your body with better choices that help burn fat efficiently.

By the end of this challenge, you'll feel stronger, more confident, and proud of the changes you've made.

Looking for Belly Fat-Burning Alternatives?

Try These Instead!

Reducing belly fat isn't just about looking better—it's about improving overall health, energy levels, and longevity. While spot-reducing fat isn't possible, smart food swaps, movement, and lifestyle changes can help you shed excess fat and build a stronger core. Use these alternatives to replace unhealthy habits and make real progress this month.

If You Crave… Try This Instead!

Sugary & Processed Carbs… Whole, Nutrient-Dense Choices
- Swap white bread and refined grains for whole wheat, quinoa, or brown rice to avoid blood sugar spikes.
- Replace sugary cereals with oatmeal topped with nuts and berries for a fiber-rich start to your day.
- Choose sweet potatoes instead of white potatoes for sustained energy without the crash.
- Replace pasta with zucchini noodles, spaghetti squash, or whole-grain alternatives.

Sugary Drinks & Alcohol… Metabolism-Boosting Alternatives
- Replace soda and juice with infused water, herbal tea, or sparkling water with lemon.
- Swap alcohol for kombucha, coconut water, or a refreshing homemade mocktail.
- Instead of energy drinks, go for green tea or black coffee for a natural metabolism boost.
- Cut back on artificial creamers and sugary lattes—try black coffee or almond milk instead.

High-Calorie Snacks… Satisfying, Protein-Rich Options
- Choose Greek yogurt with cinnamon and nuts instead of flavored yogurts with added sugar.
- Swap potato chips for air-popped popcorn, roasted chickpeas, or almonds.
- Replace candy bars with dark chocolate (70% cacao or higher) and a handful of nuts.
- Instead of granola bars, opt for homemade energy bites made with oats, nut butter, and seeds.

Late-Night Cravings… Fat-Burning & Hormone-Friendly Choices
- Replace ice cream with frozen banana slices blended with cacao powder.
- Swap late-night junk food for a protein shake or warm almond milk with cinnamon.
- Avoid mindless snacking by drinking herbal tea or lemon water to curb cravings.
- If you need something savory, go for hummus with veggies or a boiled egg instead of chips.

Sedentary Time… Movement & Strength-Building
- Replace long periods of sitting with 5-minute movement breaks every hour (stretching, squats, or planks).
- Swap mindless scrolling or TV time for a 10-minute walk after meals to help digestion.
- Instead of skipping workouts, aim for quick core-focused exercises like planks or Russian twists.
- Trade long, steady-state cardio for high-intensity interval training (HIIT) for more fat burn.

Journaling Prompts
SEPTEMBER

1 What small changes have you made to your diet or exercise routine to target belly fat?

_____

_____

_____

_____

_____

2 How does focusing on core exercises make you feel stronger or more confident?

_____

_____

_____

_____

_____

3 What non-scale victories have you noticed during this challenge?

_____

_____

_____

_____

Tighten & Tone:
Your Core Progress Tracker

This 30-day challenge is designed to help you strengthen your core and reduce belly fat through daily, targeted exercises. Use this log to record each workout, track reps or plank times, and reflect on your progress. As the month goes on, you'll build endurance, tone your midsection, and notice improvements in strength. Stick with it, and watch your core transform!

Feel free to copy this page to track additional weeks and continue your progress.

Date	Core Exercise	Sets/Reps or Time	Difficulty Level (1-5)	Notes (Energy, Progress, Adjustments)
9/1	Plank	30 seconds	**3** - Moderate	Shaky but completed it!

5 - Very Challenging **4** - Challenging **3** - Moderate **2** - Easy **1** - Very Easy

October

No Sugar Challenge

Break free from sugar addiction and experience its benefits. This chapter explains the science behind sugar cravings, suggests alternatives, and guides you through detoxing from added sugars.

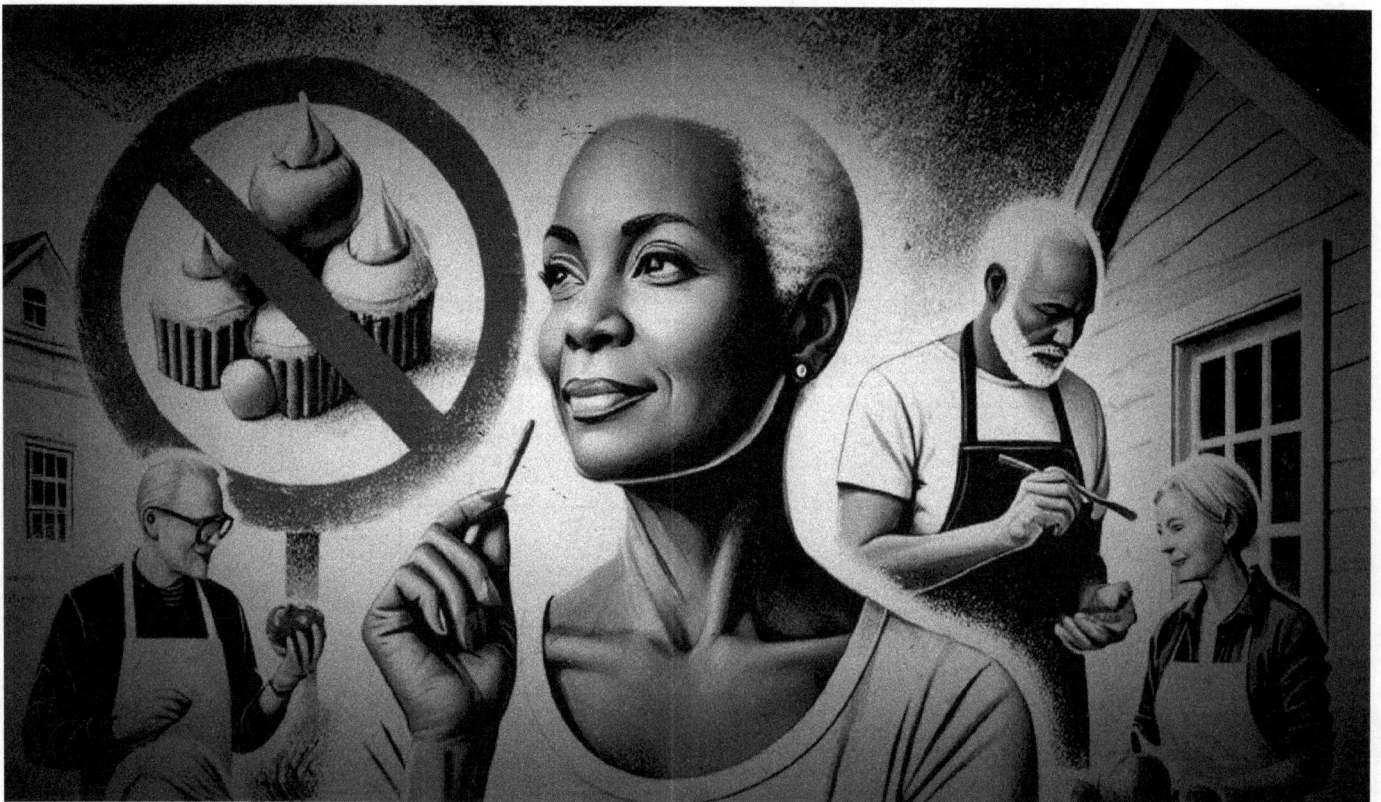

From Challenge to Change:
Real Participant Experiences

Real transformation happens when we take small, consistent steps toward better health. Each month, we challenge ourselves to build new habits, embrace positive changes, and support one another on this journey. But don't just take our word for it—hear from someone who has experienced the benefits firsthand. This testimonial highlights the real impact of this challenge and how it has helped others improve their well-being.

"For years, I'd battled with my weight—endless diets, fasting (or as I call it, starving myself), and constant guilt. Nothing worked long-term. Then I discovered the Dr. Fitness No Sugar Challenge, and for the first time, I truly understood the grip sugar had on my life. I wasn't just someone with a sweet tooth—I was a sugar addict.
The challenge opened my eyes to the hidden sugars everywhere, from "healthy" snacks to everyday condiments. Writing my sugar story was eye-opening, and it forced me to confront how sugar had become a constant in my celebrations and daily life. But thanks to the strategies and support in the challenge, I was able to reduce my cravings and identify those sneaky hidden sugars that had been sabotaging my progress.

The results have been remarkable. Cutting out sugar didn't just help me stabilize my weight—it also transformed my health. My digestion has improved, my energy levels are steady, and my mind feels clearer. Even my skin has benefited, with fewer breakouts. And knowing I'm protecting myself from chronic diseases like heart disease and diabetes is invaluable.

I'll admit, the road hasn't been easy, but I feel better than I have in years. I'm officially a recovering sugar addict, and for the first time, I know I'm not alone. If you're struggling like I was, I can't recommend the No Sugar Challenge enough. It's not just about cutting out sweets—it's about giving your body a chance to reset and thrive.

Thank you, Dr. Fitness, for this life-changing program!"

– John, Recovering Sugar Addict

Breaking Free from Sugar: A 30-Day Reset for Your Health

Sugar is everywhere—hidden in processed foods, drinks, condiments, and even so-called "healthy" snacks. While a little sugar here and there might seem harmless, excessive consumption is linked to weight gain, fatigue, inflammation, and increased risk of chronic diseases. The No Sugar Challenge isn't just about avoiding sweets—it's about giving your body a reset, stabilizing blood sugar, and experiencing what life feels like without constant sugar spikes and crashes.

1. Stabilizing Blood Sugar for Lasting Energy
One of the biggest downsides of sugar is its impact on blood sugar levels. High-sugar foods cause rapid spikes, followed by inevitable crashes, leaving you feeling sluggish and craving more sugar. Removing sugar from your diet helps your body maintain steady energy levels, reducing fatigue and brain fog.

2. Curbing Cravings and Resetting Taste Buds
Sugar is addictive—it triggers dopamine in the brain, making you crave more. The more sugar you eat, the harder it is to resist. After a few weeks without sugar, your taste buds will reset, and you'll begin to appreciate the natural sweetness of whole foods like fruits, nuts, and vegetables.

3. Supporting Weight Loss Without Counting Calories
Sugar contributes to weight gain not just because of empty calories, but because of how it triggers insulin resistance, making fat loss more difficult. Cutting out sugar helps regulate hormones, making it easier for your body to burn fat and maintain a healthy weight naturally.

4. Improving Digestion and Gut Health
Sugar feeds harmful gut bacteria, leading to bloating, digestive discomfort, and imbalances in the microbiome. When you cut sugar, you give your gut a chance to heal, improving digestion, reducing bloating, and supporting a healthier gut environment.

5. Clearer Skin and a More Youthful Glow
Excess sugar accelerates aging by breaking down collagen and elastin, leading to wrinkles and dull skin. Many people who quit sugar notice brighter, clearer skin and fewer breakouts within just a few weeks, thanks to reduced inflammation and better hydration.

6. Enhancing Mental Clarity and Mood Stability
Sugar highs and crashes don't just affect your body—they impact your brain. Too much sugar can contribute to anxiety, mood swings, and difficulty concentrating. Removing sugar helps balance neurotransmitters, leading to improved focus, stable emotions, and a clearer mind.

7. Reducing the Risk of Chronic Diseases
Excess sugar consumption is linked to an increased risk of heart disease, type 2 diabetes, and even Alzheimer's. Cutting back on sugar helps lower inflammation, improve insulin sensitivity, and support long-term health and disease prevention.

Final Thoughts: A Transformative Reset for Mind and Body
The No Sugar Challenge isn't about deprivation—it's about empowerment. It's a chance to see how your body feels when it's free from sugar's highs and lows. By the end of this challenge, you'll likely experience better energy, fewer cravings, and a deeper understanding of how sugar affects your health.

Are you ready to take control of your health and experience the benefits of a sugar-free life? Your future self will thank you!

SMART *Goals*

Write your overall goal for this month's challenge.
- **S**pecific: What exactly will you do?
- **M**easurable: How will you track your progress?
- **A**chievable: How can you realistically achieve this goal?
- **R**elevant: Why does this goal matter to you?
- **T**ime-Bound: What is the timeframe?

_____

_____

_____

_____

_____

_____

_____

_____

_____

_____

_____

_____

_____

October is a sweet reminder to say goodbye to sugar! The 30-Day No Sugar Challenge focuses on removing added sugars from your diet to improve energy, reduce cravings, and enhance overall health.

Why Take the No Sugar Challenge?

Break the Sugar Habit and Feel Better

From the Inside Out

Added sugars are linked to several health issues. Eliminating them can:

- Stabilize energy levels and mood.
- Improve sleep quality and mental clarity.
- Reduce inflammation and risk of chronic illnesses.
- Support weight loss and healthy digestion.

Tips for Success

1. Read Labels Carefully: Look for hidden sugars in packaged foods, such as condiments, bread, and sauces.
2. Use Natural Sweeteners: Replace refined sugar with small amounts of honey, dates, or maple syrup if necessary.
3. Prepare Meals at Home: Cooking your meals ensures control over ingredients and avoids hidden sugars.
4. Snack Wisely: Choose naturally sweet options like fresh fruit or unsweetened yogurt.

Common Pitfalls and How to Overcome Them

- Cravings: Distract yourself with a walk or drink herbal tea to curb sugar cravings.
- Social Events: Offer to bring a healthy dish to gatherings to ensure you have a sugar-free option.
- Low Energy: Focus on balanced meals with protein and healthy fats to maintain steady energy levels.

Sample Daily Action Plan

- Morning: Have a sugar-free breakfast like avocado toast or a veggie-packed omelet.
- Afternoon: Snack on mixed nuts or apple slices with almond butter.
- Evening: Prepare a satisfying dinner with lean protein, whole grains, and greens.

By the end of October, you'll feel lighter, more energized, and free from sugar cravings. With improved digestion, steady energy levels, and a clearer mind, you'll be equipped to make healthier choices and sustain your progress long-term.

October

- Sugar isn't just in candy—it's hidden everywhere. This challenge helps you take back control of what you eat.
- Your taste buds will change. Natural foods will taste sweeter the longer you avoid added sugar.
- Cravings don't mean you're weak—they're temporary. Drink water, eat healthy fats, or distract yourself when they hit.
- Less sugar, more energy. Cutting sugar helps prevent energy crashes, brain fog, and cravings.

Encouragement & Mindset Shift

Sugar cravings are strong, but you're stronger. This challenge helps you break the sugar addiction, stabilize your energy, and reset your taste buds for long-term health.

- Your Taste Buds Will Change – After a few weeks, natural foods will taste sweeter, and processed sweets won't be as appealing.
- Cravings Are Just a Habit – Sugar cravings usually fade after 10-15 minutes. Try drinking water or eating protein to curb the urge.
- Less Sugar, More Energy – Cutting sugar means fewer crashes, less brain fog, and more steady energy.
- Hidden Sugars Are Everywhere – Read labels and choose whole foods over processed ones.
- You're Not Giving Up Sweetness —You're Finding Healthier Ways to Enjoy It – Swap refined sugar for honey, dates, or naturally sweet foods like fruit.

By the end of this challenge, you'll feel lighter, more energetic, and in control of your cravings!

Looking for Sugar-Free Alternatives?

Try These Instead!

Cutting out sugar is one of the most transformative things you can do for your health. Excess sugar leads to energy crashes, cravings, weight gain, and inflammation—but breaking the habit doesn't mean you have to give up sweetness entirely. Try these healthy, satisfying alternatives to make the transition easier and keep cravings under control.

If You Crave... Try This Instead!

Sugary Drinks... Refreshing, Naturally Sweet Options
- Swap soda for sparkling water infused with lemon, lime, or berries.
- Replace fruit juice with water flavored with fresh orange slices or herbal tea.
- Instead of energy drinks, try green tea or black coffee for a natural caffeine boost.
- Ditch flavored coffee creamers for unsweetened almond milk and cinnamon.

Candy & Sweets... Naturally Sweet Snacks
- Choose dark chocolate (70%+ cacao) instead of milk chocolate or candy bars.
- Replace gummy candies with frozen grapes or dried fruit (unsweetened).
- Instead of caramel or chocolate sauce, drizzle nut butter or blended dates over snacks.
- Try homemade energy bites with oats, coconut, and nuts for a sweet fix.

Breakfast Cereals & Pastries... Fiber-Rich, Low-Sugar Swaps
- Swap sugary cereals for oatmeal topped with nuts, cinnamon, and berries.
- Choose plain Greek yogurt with fresh fruit instead of flavored yogurts.
- Replace muffins and pastries with whole grain toast and almond butter.
- Instead of syrup-covered pancakes, make banana pancakes topped with nut butter.

Desserts... Healthier, Low-Sugar Treats
- Freeze banana slices and blend them for a creamy ice cream alternative.
- Choose chia pudding with vanilla and unsweetened coconut milk instead of pudding cups.
- Replace cake and brownies with baked apples sprinkled with cinnamon.
- Try homemade fruit sorbet by blending frozen berries with a splash of lemon juice.

Sauces & Condiments... Hidden Sugar-Free Replacements
- Swap ketchup for mashed avocado or homemade salsa.
- Choose mustard, hummus, or guacamole instead of sugar-laden dressings.
- Replace bottled marinades with olive oil, lemon juice, and herbs.
- Opt for natural peanut or almond butter without added sugar.

Late-Night Sugar Cravings... Satisfying, Sugar-Free Fixes
- Replace ice cream with plain Greek yogurt and cinnamon.
- Sip chamomile or cinnamon tea to curb nighttime sweet cravings.
- Instead of sugary granola bars, grab a handful of nuts or pumpkin seeds.
- If you need something crunchy, try air-popped popcorn with a pinch of cinnamon.

Journaling Prompts
OCTOBER

1 What sugary foods or drinks do you miss the most, and how have you handled cravings?

_____

_____

_____

_____

2 How does eliminating sugar affect your energy levels, mood, or digestion?

_____

_____

_____

_____

3 What are three naturally sweet alternatives you've enjoyed this month?

_____

_____

_____

_____

Sweet Success: 30-Day No Sugar Tracker

Reducing sugar is one of the best things you can do for your health, energy, and mental clarity! Use this tracker to log your daily sugar-free wins, note cravings and what triggered them, and track the natural alternatives that helped. Each day, reflect on how you feel and celebrate your progress. By the end of 30 days, you'll be amazed at how much better you feel without added sugar!

Feel free to copy this page to track additional weeks and continue your progress.

Date	Sugar Free Today?	When Did The Craving Hit?	What Triggered It?	Alternative Used?	Notes (Energy, Mood, Digestion)
10/1	✔	3:00 p.m.	Afternoon slump	Apple slices w/ almond butter	Felt energized after - no crash

November

MOVEmber - 30-Day Movement Challenge

November is the perfect time to embrace movement and celebrate what your body can do. The 30-Day MOVEmber Challenge encourages you to incorporate daily movement into your routine—whether it's walking, stretching, strength training, or dancing. This challenge is about progress, not perfection, and finding ways to move that feel good to you.

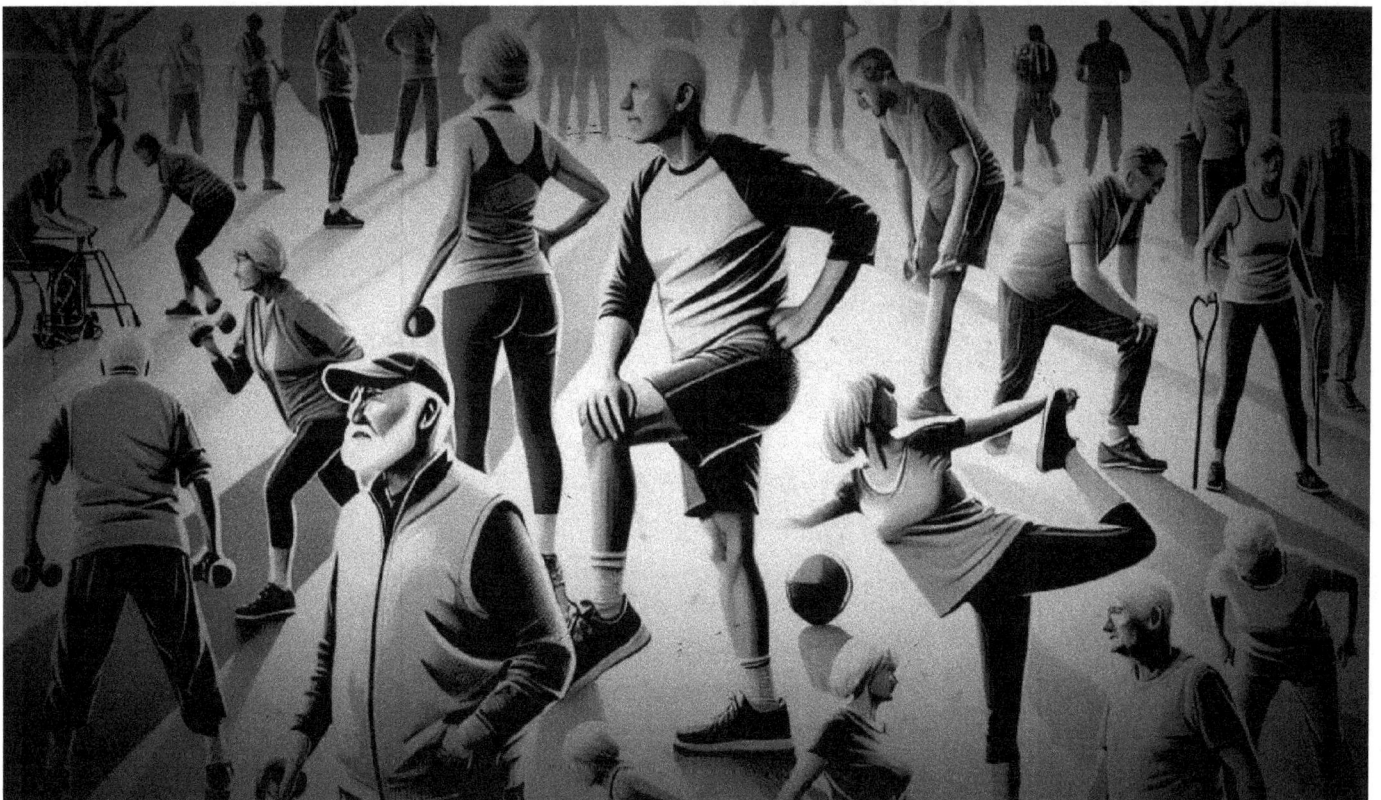

From Challenge to Change: Real Participant Experiences

Real transformation happens when we take small, consistent steps toward better health. Each month, we challenge ourselves to build new habits, embrace positive changes, and support one another on this journey. But don't just take our word for it—hear from someone who has experienced the benefits firsthand. This testimonial highlights the real impact of this challenge and how it has helped others improve their well-being.

Before joining the Dr. Fitness Movember Challenge, I was incredibly nervous about exercise. As a 74-year-old living with diabetes and fibromyalgia, past attempts at physical activity always left me in unbearable pain, and over time, I stopped exercising altogether. Unfortunately, this meant my pain worsened until I had to seek medical attention. That's when I was referred to Dr. Fitness, and it changed everything.

Dr. Fitness didn't just give me a generic plan—he truly listened to me. After understanding my challenges and personal needs, he guided me in small, manageable steps. He showed me how to sit and stand in ways that wouldn't hurt my knees, turning something as simple as standing up into part of my exercise routine. He made exercise accessible for me by integrating movement into my daily life—like feeding the ducks at the park—so it never felt boring or overwhelming.

The results have been life-changing. Over the past year, I've lost 100 pounds of fat and no longer need my diabetes medication. My blood sugar is consistently too low to require it, which has been a huge milestone for me. The biggest benefit, though, has been regaining my balance and overcoming my fear of falling. For the first time in years, I feel confident and steady on my feet.

The Dr. Fitness Movember Challenge taught me how to move safely and effectively, and for that, I'll always be grateful. Thank you, Dr. Fitness, for giving me the tools to change my life!

—Sarah 74yo, wife, mother, grandmother

MOVEember: How Daily Movement Transforms Your Body and Mind

In today's modern world, many of us spend too much time sitting—at desks, in cars, or on the couch. But movement is essential for health, not just for physical fitness but for mental clarity, longevity, and overall well-being. The MOVEmber Challenge is about incorporating movement into your daily life in a way that feels fun, sustainable, and energizing. Whether it's walking, stretching, dancing, or strength training, consistent movement has profound benefits that extend far beyond exercise.

1. Boosts Energy and Reduces Fatigue
Ironically, the more you move, the more energy you have. Physical activity increases circulation, delivering oxygen and nutrients to your cells, which helps reduce sluggishness and improve overall vitality. Even light movement, like a short walk or stretching session, can provide an instant energy boost.

2. Supports Heart Health and Longevity
Regular movement strengthens the heart, improves blood flow, and reduces the risk of heart disease. Studies show that even moderate daily activity—like brisk walking—can significantly improve cardiovascular health and increase life expectancy.

3. Improves Flexibility and Reduces Aches and Pains
Sitting for long periods can lead to stiffness, tight muscles, and poor posture. Incorporating movement throughout the day helps keep joints flexible, improves mobility, and reduces chronic pain—especially in the back, neck, and hips. Stretching, yoga, or even simple mobility exercises can make a huge difference.

4. Enhances Mental Health and Reduces Stress
Movement is one of the best natural stress relievers. Physical activity releases endorphins, the body's feel-good hormones, which can reduce anxiety and depression. Whether it's a dance session, a nature walk, or a workout, movement helps clear the mind and improve emotional well-being.

5. Strengthens Muscles and Supports Metabolism
Regular movement helps build and maintain muscle mass, which is key to supporting a healthy metabolism. Stronger muscles also mean better posture, improved balance, and a reduced risk of injuries. Strength training, bodyweight exercises, or even carrying groceries can contribute to muscle health.

6. Aids Digestion and Supports Gut Health
Movement helps stimulate digestion and prevents bloating by promoting healthy gut motility. Light activities like walking after meals can improve digestion and reduce discomfort, making movement a simple yet powerful tool for gut health.

7. Makes Exercise a Lifestyle, Not a Chore
MOVEmber isn't about rigid workouts—it's about finding joy in movement. Whether you dance while cooking, take the stairs instead of the elevator, or try a new activity like hiking or swimming, movement should feel enjoyable and natural. The more fun you have with movement, the more likely you are to keep it a lifelong habit.

Final Thoughts: A Month to Build Lasting Habits
MOVEmber is an invitation to embrace movement in all forms and discover how even small changes can lead to big improvements in your health. By the end of the challenge, you'll feel more energized, flexible, and connected to your body. The goal isn't perfection—it's consistency, enjoyment, and making movement a part of your daily routine.

Are you ready to move more, feel better, and build habits that last beyond November? Let's get moving!

SMART *Goals*

Write your overall goal for this month's challenge.
- **S**pecific: What exactly will you do?
- **M**easurable: How will you track your progress?
- **A**chievable: How can you realistically achieve this goal?
- **R**elevant: Why does this goal matter to you?
- **T**ime-Bound: What is the timeframe?

_____

_____

_____

_____

_____

_____

_____

_____

_____

_____

_____

_____

November is the perfect time to embrace movement and celebrate what your body can do. The 30-Day MOVEmber Challenge encourages you to incorporate daily movement into your routine—whether it's walking, stretching, strength training, or dancing. This challenge is about progress, not perfection, and finding ways to move that feel good to you.

Embrace Movement
And Celebrate What Your Body Can Do

Why Take the MOVEmber Challenge?

Regular movement has profound benefits, including:

- Boosting mood and reducing stress by releasing endorphins.
- Strengthening muscles and improving flexibility.
- Enhancing cardiovascular health and endurance.
- Increasing energy levels and promoting better sleep.
- Supporting overall well-being and longevity.

Tips for Success

1. Start Where You Are: Whether you're a beginner or experienced, tailor movement to your fitness level.
2. Make It Fun: Choose activities you enjoy, like dancing, hiking, or yoga.
3. Incorporate Movement Throughout the Day: Walk during phone calls, take the stairs, or stretch during breaks.
4. Set Realistic Goals: Aim for at least 30 minutes of movement per day, but listen to your body.
5. Track Your Progress: Keep a log of your daily movement and how you feel.

Common Pitfalls and How to Overcome Them

- Lack of Motivation: Find a workout buddy or playlist that gets you excited to move.
- Time Constraints: Break movement into smaller chunks throughout the day.
- Body Aches or Stiffness: Start with gentle stretching or low-impact activities like walking or swimming.
- Boredom: Switch up your workouts, try new activities, or set movement challenges.

Sample Daily Action Plan

- Morning: Stretch for 5–10 minutes to wake up your body.
- Afternoon: Take a 10-minute walk or do bodyweight exercises.
- Evening: Engage in a fun activity like dancing, yoga, or cycling.

November

- Movement is a Powerhouse. Moving your body daily strengthens muscles, improves circulation, and boosts overall vitality.
- This is about adding, not pushing. The more you move, the more your body will crave activity and reward you with increased energy and flexibility.
- You'll feel the benefits fast. Better mood, improved endurance, and reduced stiffness can happen within days.
- Movement doesn't have to be boring. Experiment with different activities—dance, stretch, hike, lift, or even just take the stairs—to keep it fresh and exciting!

Encouragement & Mindset Shift

Movement isn't just about exercise—it's about celebrating what your body can do. This challenge isn't about pushing yourself to extremes; it's about integrating movement into your daily life in ways that feel good and sustainable.

- Movement Is Medicine – A little movement each day can improve mental and physical health.
- Small Steps Matter – Even five extra minutes of movement can boost energy and mood.
- Listen to Your Body – Move in ways that feel good and respect your limits.
- Find Joy in Motion – Choose activities that bring you happiness and fulfillment.
- This Is a Lifestyle Shift – By the end of the challenge, moving your body will feel natural and rewarding.

Looking for ways to stay active?

Try these movement ideas throughout the month:

If You Love Structure, Try:
- Yoga or Pilates
- Strength training circuits
- Walking or running programs
- Fitness classes (online or in-person)

If You Enjoy Fun & Play, Try:
- Dancing to your favorite music
- Hiking or exploring nature
- Jump rope or hula hoop
- Playing sports or active games

If You Need Stress Relief, Try:
- Tai chi or Qigong
- Stretching or mobility drills
- Deep breathing with movement
- Gentle evening walks

If You Have Limited Time, Try:
- 10-minute bodyweight exercises
- Taking the stairs instead of the elevator
- Parking farther away and walking more
- Desk stretches and chair yoga

If You Want to Build Strength, Try:
- Bodyweight exercises (push-ups, squats, lunges)
- Resistance band training
- Functional fitness (lifting groceries, carrying kids, housework with intention)
- Kettlebell swings or dumbbell training

If You Like a Challenge, Try:
- A 30-day plank or squat challenge
- Interval running or HIIT workouts
- Climbing stairs or doing hill sprints
- Practicing a new skill like handstands or jump rope tricks

Journaling Prompts
MOVEMBER

1 How does daily movement impact your energy, mood, and focus?

_____

_____

_____

_____

2 What type of movement brings you the most joy, and how can you do more of it?

_____

_____

_____

_____

3 How can movement become a lifelong habit rather than a temporary challenge?

_____

_____

_____

_____

MOVEmber:
30-Day Movement Tracker

Use this tracker to log your daily movement and reflect on how it makes you feel. By the end of the challenge, you'll have a record of your progress and insights into how movement benefits your life.

Feel free to copy this page to track additional weeks and continue your progress.

Date	Type of Movement	Duration	How I Felt Before & Aafter
11/1	Walking	15 minutes	Was resistant to going for a walk but felt energized after I did.

December

No Fast Food Challenge

End the year strong by cooking at home and skipping fast food. Learn simple recipes, time-saving cooking hacks, and how to balance convenience with health.

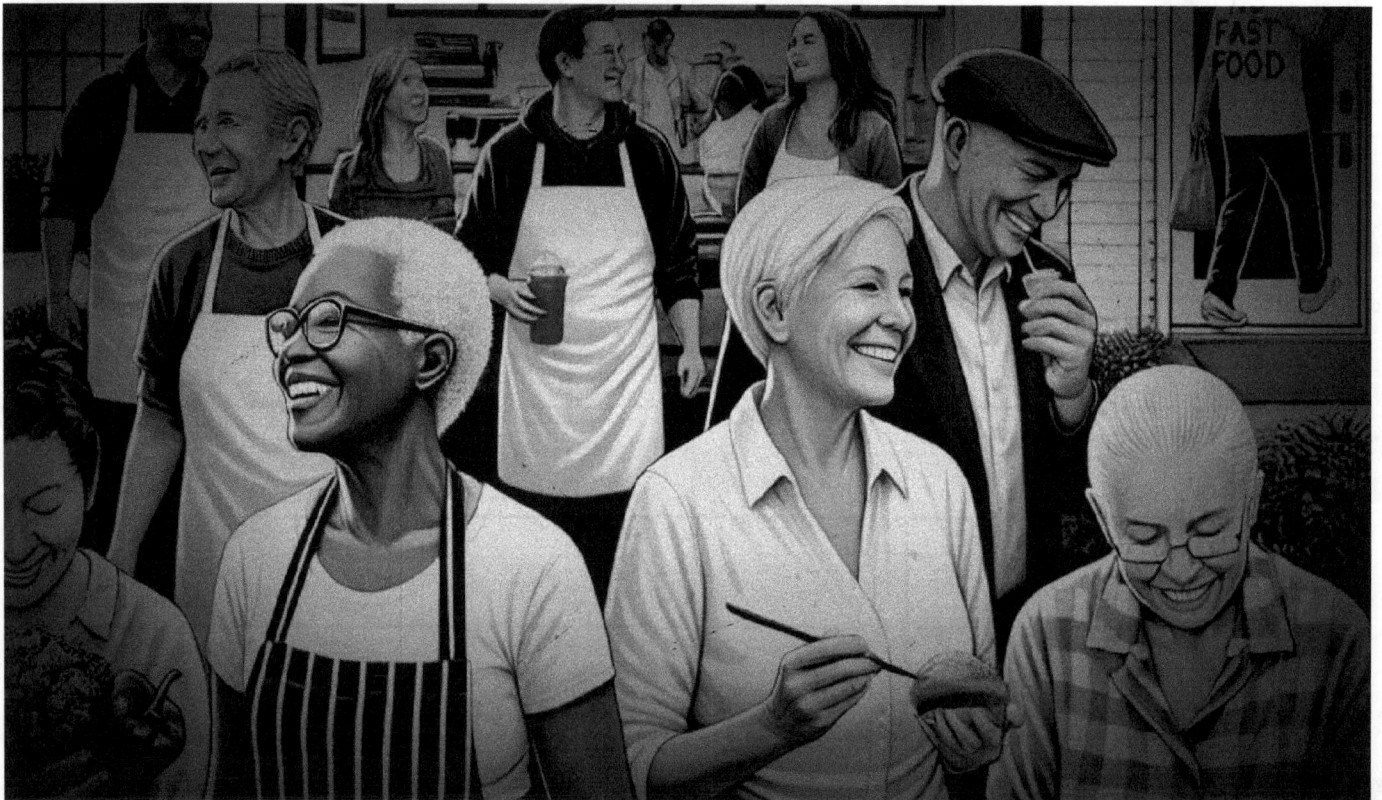

From Challenge to Change: Real Participant Experiences

Real transformation happens when we take small, consistent steps toward better health. Each month, we challenge ourselves to build new habits, embrace positive changes, and support one another on this journey. But don't just take our word for it—hear from someone who has experienced the benefits firsthand. This testimonial highlights the real impact of this challenge and how it has helped others improve their well-being.

"Last December was a turning point for my family, thanks to the '30 Day No Fast Food Challenge.' As a single dad with two pre-teen daughters, I relied heavily on fast food—it was quick and convenient after long workdays. But then we heard Dr. Fitness on 93.3 The Beat Jamz, challenging listeners to give up fast food for the month of December. His message about how fast food habits contribute to childhood obesity struck a chord with me. I realized I needed to make a change, not just for myself but for my girls, who were struggling with their weight.

We decided to take the challenge, and I couldn't have done it without the support provided. Dr. Fitness sent us easy, no-cook recipes that were healthy, fast, and surprisingly delicious. He even recommended prepared meal options that were just as affordable as fast food but a lot healthier. Over the 30 days, we not only resisted our usual holiday weight gain but actually lost belly fat and felt more energetic. My daughters and I also learned a lot about food preparation, and I realized that eating healthy doesn't have to be hard or time-consuming.

This experience was life-changing. We no longer fear healthy eating, and our small lifestyle change has improved our health and bonded us as a family. I'm so grateful to Dr. Fitness for helping us break the fast food cycle."

— David, single dad of two pre-teens

Breaking the Fast Food Habit: A 30-Day Challenge for Healthier Eating

Fast food is convenient, cheap, and everywhere—but at what cost? While grabbing a quick meal on the go might seem harmless, fast food is often packed with unhealthy fats, excessive sodium, added sugars, and preservatives that can take a serious toll on your health. The No Fast Food Challenge is about taking back control of your nutrition, choosing real, whole foods, and experiencing the incredible benefits of home-cooked meals.

1. Eliminating Hidden Calories and Processed Ingredients
Fast food is designed to be hyper-palatable, meaning it's loaded with artificial flavors, excessive salt, and unhealthy fats to keep you coming back for more. Cutting it out for 30 days eliminates these hidden additives, helping your body function more efficiently and reducing cravings for processed foods.

2. Improved Digestion and Reduced Bloating
Fast food meals are often low in fiber and high in refined ingredients that can slow digestion and cause bloating. By replacing processed meals with whole foods, you support gut health, improve digestion, and reduce stomach discomfort.

3. More Stable Energy Levels and Fewer Crashes
The combination of refined carbs and added sugars in fast food can send blood sugar levels soaring—only to crash soon after, leaving you feeling sluggish and craving more unhealthy food. When you switch to real, nutrient-dense meals, your energy stays stable throughout the day.

4. Supporting Heart Health and Lowering Inflammation
Regular consumption of fast food is linked to higher cholesterol, increased blood pressure, and systemic inflammation. By eliminating it, you allow your body to heal, reducing the risk of heart disease and supporting long-term cardiovascular health.

5. Weight Management Without Restrictive Dieting
Fast food is calorie-dense but nutrient-poor, making it easy to overeat without feeling satisfied. By switching to homemade meals, you naturally regulate portion sizes, consume more fiber and protein, and support healthy weight management—without the need for extreme dieting.

6. Saving Money While Eating Better
Fast food might seem like a budget-friendly option, but the costs add up over time. Cooking at home allows you to stretch your grocery budget further while enjoying higher-quality, healthier meals. Plus, meal prepping helps reduce food waste and makes eating healthy even more convenient.

7. Building Long-Term Healthy Habits
This challenge isn't about never eating fast food again—it's about developing a better relationship with food. By the end of 30 days, you'll likely find that home-cooked meals are more satisfying, flavorful, and nourishing than anything from a drive-thru. Learning to prepare simple, nutritious meals sets the foundation for a lifetime of healthier eating choices.

Final Thoughts: A Reset for Your Body and Mind
The No Fast Food Challenge is an opportunity to break the cycle of unhealthy eating and experience how great your body feels when fueled by real, whole foods. By the end of this challenge, you'll have more energy, improved digestion, and a greater appreciation for home-cooked meals.

Are you ready to ditch fast food and embrace healthier, more nourishing choices? Your body—and your future self—will thank you!

SMART *Goals*

Write your overall goal for this month's challenge.
- **S**pecific: What exactly will you do?
- **M**easurable: How will you track your progress?
- **A**chievable: How can you realistically achieve this goal?
- **R**elevant: Why does this goal matter to you?
- **T**ime-Bound: What is the timeframe?

_____

_____

_____

_____

_____

_____

_____

_____

_____

_____

_____

_____

_____

December can be a hectic month, filled with holiday parties, shopping, and family gatherings. The 30-Day No Fast Food Challenge helps you end the year on a healthy note by avoiding fast food and prioritizing home-cooked meals.

Finish the Year Strong With

Home-Cooked Meals

Why Take the No Fast Food Challenge?

Steering clear of fast food can:

- Improve overall nutrition by focusing on wholesome, home-prepared meals.
- Save money by cutting out costly fast food stops.
- Reduce intake of unhealthy fats, sodium, and empty calories.
- Strengthen family bonds through shared meal preparation.
- Encourage mindfulness about what you're eating.

Tips for Success

- Plan Ahead: Prepare meals and snacks in advance to avoid last-minute fast food runs.
- Explore New Recipes: Get creative with healthy, easy-to-make dishes at home.
- Pack Your Meals: Bring homemade lunches and snacks to work or when running errands.
- Keep It Simple: Focus on quick, nutritious meals like stir-fries, soups, and roasted vegetables.

Common Pitfalls and How to Overcome Them

- Time Constraints: Use a slow cooker or instant pot to save time on meal prep.
- Temptation: Keep healthy snacks in your bag or car to avoid stopping for fast food.
- Holiday Parties: Eat a small, healthy meal beforehand so you're not overly hungry when surrounded by indulgent options.

Sample Daily Action Plan

- *Morning:* Start your day with a nutritious homemade breakfast—try oatmeal with nuts and berries, a smoothie with protein and greens, or eggs with whole-grain toast.
- *Afternoon:* Pack a healthy, satisfying lunch—like a quinoa salad, grilled chicken wrap, or homemade soup—to take to work or on errands.
- Keep a stash of easy, nutritious snacks (like mixed nuts, hummus with veggies, or a hard-boiled egg) to prevent hunger-driven fast-food temptations.
- *Evening:* Prepare a balanced home-cooked dinner—choose a simple recipe like stir-fried vegetables with lean protein, a grain bowl, or a hearty soup.
- Set aside leftovers for lunch the next day, making it easier to stick to the challenge.

By the end of December, you'll have transformed your eating habits, gained confidence in meal planning, and discovered the joy of nourishing your body with wholesome, home-cooked meals. With improved energy, better digestion, and a deeper awareness of your food choices, you'll step into the new year feeling empowered, healthier, and more in control of your well-being.

December

- Fast food is designed to be addictive. Breaking the cycle frees you from cravings and unhealthy habits.
- Meal prep is your secret weapon. When you have healthy food ready, fast food isn't tempting.
- Your body will feel the difference. Fewer processed foods mean less bloating, better digestion, and more energy.
- This is about long-term change, not just one month. Learning to cook and choose better options will benefit you for life.

Encouragement & Mindset Shift

Fast food is designed to be cheap, convenient, and addictive—but you have the power to break the cycle and take back control of your meals.

- Fast Food Doesn't Mean Fast Health – It often leads to fatigue, bloating, and nutrient deficiencies.
- You're Gaining More Than You're Giving Up – More energy, better digestion, and fewer cravings are worth it.
- Meal Prep Is Your Best Friend – Having homemade meals ready makes it easier to avoid drive-thrus.
- Your Wallet Will Thank You – Cooking at home saves money while improving your health.
- You'll Feel More in Control – This challenge isn't just about food—it's about making mindful choices every day.

By the end of this challenge, you'll feel lighter, more energized, and in control of your eating habits!

Looking for Fast Food Alternatives?

Try These Instead!

Fast food is convenient, but it often comes with excess calories, unhealthy fats, and added sugars that leave you feeling sluggish. This challenge helps you break the fast-food habit by replacing it with nutritious, homemade meals that are just as satisfying. Use these smart swaps to enjoy quick, healthy options without the drive-thru.

If You Crave... Try This Instead!

Fast-Food Breakfast... Quick & Healthy Morning Options
- A homemade breakfast sandwich with whole grain toast, eggs, and avocado instead of a drive-thru biscuit.
- Overnight oats with nuts, berries, and almond milk instead of sugary breakfast pastries.
- Greek yogurt with granola and honey instead of a fast-food parfait.
- A protein smoothie with banana, peanut butter, and spinach instead of a high-calorie coffee drink.

Greasy Burgers & Fried Foods... Satisfying Homemade Alternatives
- A homemade turkey or black bean burger on a whole wheat bun instead of a fast-food burger.
- Air-fried sweet potato fries instead of greasy French fries.
- Baked chicken tenders with almond flour coating instead of fried chicken.
- Grilled chicken with brown rice and steamed veggies instead of a fast-food combo meal.

Pizza & Takeout... Easy, Healthier Swaps
- Whole wheat pita pizza with tomato sauce and veggies instead of delivery pizza.
- Cauliflower crust pizza instead of a deep-dish or stuffed crust.
- Stir-fried tofu or chicken with brown rice instead of greasy takeout Chinese food.
- Homemade taco bowls with black beans and avocado instead of fast-food tacos.

Sugary Drinks & Shakes... Refreshing, Low-Sugar Choices
- Herbal tea or flavored sparkling water instead of soda.
- Iced coffee with almond milk instead of a sugar-loaded Frappuccino.
- A homemade smoothie with banana and cacao powder instead of a milkshake.
- Coconut water with a squeeze of lime instead of sweetened sports drinks.

Late-Night Fast Food Cravings... Easy, Homemade Fixes
- Whole grain toast with almond butter instead of a drive-thru dessert.
- A protein bar or nuts instead of a fast-food snack.
- Popcorn with olive oil and sea salt instead of fries.
- A hard-boiled egg with veggies instead of late-night nachos.

Journaling Prompts
DECEMBER

1 What are the biggest obstacles you've faced in avoiding fast food, and how have you overcome them?

_____

_____

_____

_____

_____

2 How do homemade meals compare to fast food in terms of taste, cost, and nutrition?

_____

_____

_____

_____

_____

3 What new cooking skills or recipes have you learned during this challenge?

_____

_____

_____

_____

Ditch the Drive-Thru: 30-Day No Fast Food Challenge

Skipping fast food isn't just about eating healthier—it's about saving money, feeling better, and learning to enjoy home-cooked meals! Use this tracker to log your daily home-prepped meals, estimate your savings, and reflect on your favorite meals each week. By the end of 30 days, you'll have built a habit of choosing nutritious, homemade food over fast food while keeping more money in your pocket!

Feel free to copy this page to track additional weeks and continue your progress.

Date	Home Cooked Meals	Estimated Savings $$	Notes (Cravings, Energy, New Recipes)
12/1	Scrambled eggs, grilled chicken salad, veggie stir fry	$15	Felt great cooking at home, no cravings!

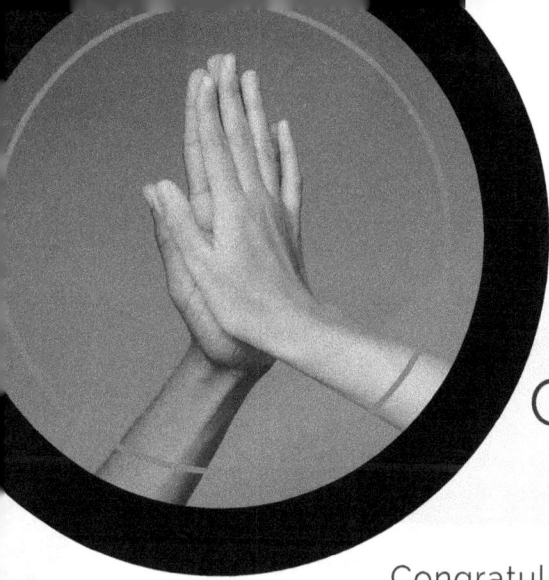

Final Reflection:
Celebrating Your Progress & Looking Ahead

Congratulations on completing this 12-month journey of small yet powerful steps toward better health and well-being! Whether you followed the challenges in order or picked and chose the ones that spoke to you most, you've taken intentional steps toward a healthier lifestyle. Now, it's time to reflect, solidify your progress, and decide what comes next.

Your Top 3 Takeaways
Think back over the past year. What were the most impactful changes you made? Which habits felt the most natural, and which required more effort? Take a moment to write down the three habits you want to continue for life:

1. _____

   _____

   _____

   _____

2. _____

   _____

   _____

   _____

3. _____

   _____

   _____

   _____

By identifying these key habits, you create a foundation for long-term wellness. These aren't just "challenges" anymore—they're part of who you are.

Maintaining Momentum: Avoiding Setbacks & Stacking Habits

Building lasting habits isn't about perfection—it's about persistence. Life happens, and setbacks are inevitable. The key is knowing how to get back on track.

How to Stay on Track

- Use Habit Stacking: Pair new habits with established ones. Example: Drink a glass of water first thing in the morning before checking your phone.

- Create Non-Negotiables: Set small daily goals that you always do, like a 5-minute stretch or a mindful deep breath session.

- Schedule Check-Ins: Once a month, reflect on how your habits are going. Adjust as needed.

- Track Your Wins: Keep a journal or app to log progress. Even minor victories add up!

- Set Visual Reminders: Place sticky notes, use phone reminders, or keep a vision board to reinforce your goals.

- Make It Enjoyable: Find ways to make your habits fun—listen to music while exercising or turn meal prep into a creative experiment.

- Reward Yourself: Celebrate small milestones with non-food rewards like a relaxing bath, a new book, or a fun outing.

What to Do If You Slip

- Be Kind to Yourself: Everyone has off days. The goal is consistency, not perfection.

- Recommit Immediately: Don't wait for a Monday or next month—restart your habit at the next opportunity.

- Adjust the Challenge: If a habit feels overwhelming, break it into smaller steps.

- Reflect on Triggers: Identify what caused the setback and develop a strategy to avoid it in the future.

- Seek Support: Reach out to a friend, mentor, or support group for encouragement and accountability.

Creating Your Personalized Habit-Building Roadmap

Now that you've built a foundation of healthier habits, it's time to personalize your journey. Use the following template to map out your next wellness goals. Your Next 30-Day Challenge:

- **Challenge Topic:** _____
  _____
  _____

- **Why This Matters to You:** _____
  _____
  _____

- **How You Will Measure Success:** _____
  _____
  _____

- **Potential Challenges & Solutions:** _____
  _____
  _____

- **Daily or Weekly Action Steps:** _____
  _____
  _____

Whether you revisit previous challenges or create new ones, your success is in your hands!

Community & Support: Stay Connected & Keep Growing

Ways to Stay Connected:
- Find a Like-Minded Community: Join online wellness groups, local fitness meetups, or virtual accountability circles. Being part of a group keeps motivation high and provides a space to ask questions, share wins, and seek support when needed.
- Accountability Partners: Team up with a friend, coach, or mentor who can check in with you regularly. Having someone to share progress with makes it easier to stay committed and work through obstacles together.
- Share Your Journey: Inspire others by documenting your progress on social media, in a personal blog, or through a wellness journal. Not only does sharing your journey keep you accountable, but it may also encourage someone else to begin their own transformation.
- Keep Learning: Growth never stops. Read books, listen to podcasts, take online courses, or attend workshops to expand your knowledge and maintain curiosity about wellness trends and practices.
- Give Back & Encourage Others: Teaching and supporting others can reinforce your own habits. Consider mentoring someone new to wellness or offering encouragement to people just starting their journey.

The Power of Revisiting This Journey

If you found this journey helpful, consider revisiting it next year. Each time you go through these challenges, you'll gain new insights, deepen your habits, and reinforce your commitment to a healthier, happier life. Habits build upon themselves, and by taking small steps every day, you are creating a foundation for lifelong wellness.

Here's to taking small steps—every single day—toward a life of vitality, balance, and joy!

Call to Action: If you'd like to continue your wellness journey with Dr. Fitness and his community, please text your name, email address, and the word CHALLENGE to 904-236-5858 to stay connected!

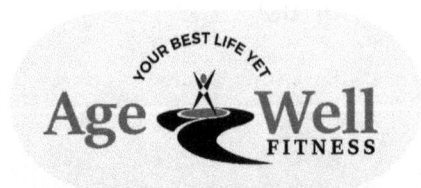

YOUR BEST LIFE YET

Age Well
FITNESS

Additional Resources

American Lung Association

The American Lung Association is a leading organization dedicated to improving lung health and preventing lung disease through research, education, and advocacy. Whether you need support to quit smoking, manage a chronic lung condition, or learn more about lung health, their resources and programs can provide valuable assistance. For more information:

800-lungusa or 1-800-586-4872
www.lung.org

Alcoholics Anonymous (AA)

Alcoholics Anonymous offers a worldwide fellowship of individuals seeking to overcome alcohol addiction through peer support and a structured recovery program. With meetings available in-person and online, AA provides a safe and judgment-free space to share experiences and receive guidance on the journey to sobriety. Learn more or find a local meeting:

212-870-3400
www.aa.org

American Cancer Society

The American Cancer Society is dedicated to fighting cancer through research, advocacy, and patient support services. From early detection and prevention to treatment guidance and survivorship programs, the ACS provides crucial resources for those affected by cancer. For assistance or more information:

800-acs-2345 or 800-227-2345
www.cancer.org

www.ingramcontent.com/pod-product-compliance
Lightning Source LLC
Chambersburg PA
CBHW050240290326
41930CB00043B/3181